ADVANCED PRAISE

I first met Crystal during the initial stages of the writing process and watched her develop her thoughts into actions, or in other words, she WALKS the TALK. I am so proud of Crystal getting her message out to lift other women. She is a modern-day warrior of self-care, which is crucial in order to be of service to others. Her raw stories of sports, sobriety, and spine surgery give all of us hope. Crystal leaves you with a feeling and belief that anything really is possible!

—Tony Mandarich
Author of *My Dirty Little Secrets - Steroids, Alcohol & God*
Sobriety Advocate & NFL Alumni

Connecting with Crystal completely changed the trajectory of my life. I had never met anyone sober before, and it was like lightning had struck me. She had so many of the things I wanted in my life but hadn't been able to achieve and I wondered if alcohol could be the culprit. She helped me to take the necessary action I needed to get to where I am today—the healthiest I have ever been, in a mindful space with alcohol, enjoying running my own business, happy in my relationships and the mother to a beautiful baby girl. Truly an inspiration to women everywhere and not only in the realm of health and fitness but in her generosity, beauty, determination and especially in her dedication to be an amazing mother. I am lucky to have her on my team as a friend and mentor.

—Candice Martina Fairorth
GoingForGoddess.com

I've suffered from back pain alongside Crystal for many years. I have also suffered from severe depression that leaves me with the question, "Has the pain caused my depression, or does depression cause my pain?" To see her pain free and thriving gives hope to anyone who has struggled with chronic life-debilitating conditions. I love that Crystal shared the journey of creating her modified low impact poses with yoga and living a natural lifestyle to manage her wellbeing without relying on medication. Her book, *Quitting to Win,* gives hope to all who suffer from back pain, alcoholism, and depression. She is a beacon of hope for me.

—Dejah Hatfield
Teammate and longtime friend

Crystal's proven path gives you the tools you need. She is a warrior of self-care. Her raw stories of sports, sobriety, and spine surgery give all those who suffer a message of hope.

—Kary Oberbrunner
Author of *Your Secret Name* and *Elixir Project*

Crystal has shown that with Jesus, anything is possible.

—Kim Dolan Leto
Author of *F.I.T Faith Inspired Transformation*

I met Crystal well into her healing. To watch her develop her thoughts into actions, has been a journey of determination fueled by a spirit of gratitude. I share Crystal's passion for getting her message out to lift and inspire other women. She is a warrior of self-care; which is so important in order to be of service to others. Her raw stories of sports, sobriety and spine surgery give all those who suffer, hope and encouragement.

—Daphne V. Smith
Author of *What's YOUR Scarlet Letter?*

Sports, something almost all of us engaged in growing up, can create a framework around which you can build a meaningful, joyous life. Crystal does a superb job in showing us how.

—George Fleming
Momentum Coaching Resources

Being Crystal's sister, I have watched as she has developed into the person she is today, living her best life by setting boundaries. I admire her spiritual fitness and her willingness to carry the message to others.

—Jessica Zaragoza
Sister

Having accompanied Crystal to many of her pre & post back surgery appointments, I saw her at a very painful low in her life. She used her Faith, Sobriety, and "Food as Fuel" knowledge to put herself "back" together. *Quitting to Win* is a must read for anyone looking for a path from pain to peace.

—Tammy Cozzi
Yoga & Faith friend

I have known Crystal for over 20 years and had a front-row seat to her journey. She is a beacon of hope to those that suffer from alcoholism/addiction.

—Annalisa Wagoner
Friend

QUITTING TO WIN

A Proven Plan to Let Go of Bad Habits, Learn to Feel, and Love Yourself

Crystal Waltman

CRYSTAL WALTMAN

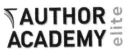

Quitting to Win
A Proven Plan to Let Go of Bad Habits,
Learn to Feel, and Love Yourself
© 2020 Crystal Waltman
All rights reserved.

Printed in the United States of America

Published by Author Academy Elite
P.O. Box 43, Powell, OH 43035
AuthorAcademyElite.com

Visit the author's website at www.crystalwaltman.com

For quantity orders or to book speaking engagements
contact us directly at
info@crystalwaltman.com

Paperback: 978-1-64746-215-4
Hardback: 978-1-64746-216-1
Ebook: 978-1-64746-217-8

Library of Congress Control Number: 2020905637

Although the author and publisher have made every effort to ensure that
the information in this book was correct at press time, the author and
publisher do not assume and herby disclaim any liability to any party for
any loss, damage or disruption caused by errors or omission, whether such
errors or omissions result from negligence, accident, or any other cause.

Unless otherwise noted, Scripture quotations are taken from the New
International Version, NIV. © 1973, 1978, 1984, 2011 by Biblica, Inc.
TM. Used by permission of Zondervan. All rights reserved worldwide.

Disclaimer

The stories in this book have been documented from the best of my memory. It is with love and respect that I acknowledge the people that have touched my life. Most of the names have been changed to protect everyone's privacy. I fondly refer to the Alcoholic Anonymous Book as The Big Book, and the Bible as The Word.

CONTENTS

DEDICATION

I dedicate this book to my daughter, Liv. May your life be filled with joy and compassion. Learn from my past—there is no need to repeat it. My redemption is in your soul. You are enough, for you are made by God. May you get your worth from *The Word*, not the world. I dedicate this book to my husband, Michael, who reminds me daily to take it easy. There is no one I would rather journey through this life with. To my stepsons, Alec and Jared, God blessed me with you two, and I would not have it any other way. I could not have put these words to paper without all of your unwavering support. For all the times I wanted to quit, and you encouraged me to keep going, I love you all so much. You are my rock, the foundation where everything begins and ends.

This book is also dedicated to the people whose lives were cut short. Instead of getting their names tattooed on my left shoulder in Old English, I decided to put the ink on paper instead and dedicate this book to them.

Scarlett Smith
1979-1997

William Prior
1949-2014

Jennifer Paisley
1963-2017

Sandy Simon
1944-2018

I also choose to share my story in hopes of helping anyone dealing with depression, eating disorders, alcoholism, and other diseases caused by lifestyle-choices. Know you are not alone.

INTRODUCTION

From the outside, it looks like my passions are health and fitness.

Since I was very young, I was taught to be physically competitive. I started playing softball at ten years old and received a college scholarship to play at the highest level. Winning a national title by nineteen, I felt so blessed to receive these honors and opportunities that playing competitive sports gifted me with.

Between the ages of twenty-five and thirty-five, I either trained for something important or overindulged in things that could take it all away. As far back as I can remember, I had based my worth on my outer appearance and performance, instead of character. This left me feeling empty and insecure. My body weight yo-yoed, and as it did, so did my feelings of self-worth. I rode on the emotional roller coaster that came with it, experiencing the rise and fall that comes with every young girl's identity. Because I could not see middle ground between the two extremes, I felt as though I was either really high or really low. Although I had even won a competition for low body fat and physical symmetry, when I held that first-place trophy, I remember thinking this can't be what health and fitness feels like. I should have felt proud and accomplished, but I still felt like something was missing.

I spent hours in the gym and also trained women one-on-one to continue my career in physical fitness. But outside of the gym, I found it hard to engage anyone in small talk. It always seemed to flow for many other women, but I came across stand-offish because that kind of connection never came naturally for me unless I had something to take the edge off.

Again, I couldn't help but feel there was always something missing. What was missing was my spiritual connection and the right intentions of inner physical and mental health. Instead of leading with my accomplishments, I find it creates a greater bond when I lead with progress. I strive for progress, not perfection. Lord knows I am not perfect by any means.

As a young adult, I couldn't picture myself past the age of forty. Surprisingly, when I made it to my fortieth birthday, I finally jumped off the emotional roller coaster. I realized the value of emotional sobriety, and I worked to strengthen and maintain my spiritual fitness. That is what drove me to write this book, because I felt if I could step outside my comfort zone to write my story, then maybe I could inspire others to work on their own spiritual fitness.

> When you work on the inside, the
> outside will follow.
>
> —Kim Dolan Leto

In the appendix of the book, I attached discussion questions to go along with each chapter. This is to help you pause and reflect on what is going on in your life to see how to reconcile the past, and live in the moment. These discussion questions are meant to be used for a small group study or book club.

PART 1

QUIT SHUTTING THE DOOR ON YOUR PAST

The stories I share with you are stories that have been buried deep inside my soul for many years. I never wanted to let anyone know this less-than-perfect part of me. Thankfully, my perspective has changed, and I choose to tell my stories. My experiences molded me into who I am today, and I am set free by sharing. If my stories help one young athlete, sexual assault victim, wife, mother, or daughter find her serenity, it is all worth it. The stories that follow are some of the moments that defined who I am today, and I share them in hopes that they might inspire you to start looking at your own.

I don't regret the past or wish to shut the door on it.

—*The Big Book*

CHAPTER 1
QUIT WISHING IT WAS YOU AND NOT THEM

SOFTBALL, SCHOLARSHIPS, AND SUICIDE

We are only as sick as our secrets.

—*The Big Book*

I t was a winter night in Phoenix, Arizona, and the skies were clear and dark with bright stars. I felt the cold air on my face and the alcohol running through my veins. The familiar scent of the mesquite smoke floated in the air from those households fortunate enough to have fireplaces. A high school best friend and I were together once again. Scarlett and I had gone to separate colleges to play softball. I always wished I was her with a doting father, a little sister who loved her, and a mom who was involved in every part of her life.

We started our winter break with laughs and hugs. A couple of compadres reunited for Christmas break at my parents' house where we shared stories about college, coaches, teammates, and boys. The zing of cocaine was warmed by shots of vodka. We shared smokes, laughs, and the light of the full moon. The night was bright and so were our futures.

As if no time had passed, we picked right back up with our partying ways. We caught up on epic events of the last few semesters. Scarlett's life was so dreamy, right out of a story book. Her parents had given her all the best opportunities and material things money could buy. We felt no pain, and we both had a good buzz going. Because we had both achieved our dreams of making it to college, we felt like we were on cloud nine. Back then, you had to make plans in person. There was no *friend finder*, *location sharing*, or last-minute *texting*. But still, we had an internal instinct that helped us find our friends at a moment's notice.

It was time for my friend to share the rest of her night with her ex-boyfriend, so I said good-bye with a warm embrace. No matter where Scarlett was, someone was missing her and waiting for her to come back. Before she left, Scarlett suggested, "Let's hang at the river bottom tomorrow night!" We smiled at each other and begrudgingly, she left.

I had agreed with a grin to meet the next night. The Sonoran Desert was our river bottom. Out there, Arizona nights were at their finest. With the closest housing development six miles away, it gave us a sense of freedom to spend time away from the world. Surrounded by peace and quiet, there was nothing but the sounds of four-wheeling trucks, country music, and the smell of burning pallets to make a bonfire. As long as we did not burn car tires, the cops rarely showed up.

"Great!" Scarlett had said. "I'll pick you up, and we can go for a day drive." She had a love for driving, whether it was her sports car, truck, or SUV. It was an escape for her—the loud music and the windows down with the wind in her hair. This gave her a sense of freedom. She took pride in her vehicles by keeping them clean, waxing them by hand in her driveway on a Sunday afternoon in jean shorts and a bikini top as she simultaneously tried to get a suntan. "See you tomorrow," I had said to Scarlett as she waved goodbye and drove out of the cul-de-sac. I was happy to see her but sad to see her go; I wished we had more time together. As she drove away, I smiled and laughed as I thought of how grown we were. I remembered all the silly things we had done, most of them involved vehicles from four-wheeling mudding to crashing a car while she was attempting to race, to submerging a vehicle, to a boat sinking. We were fearless together.

Before she headed home that night, Scarlett made one stop at a high school boyfriend's house. He was a real piece of work—violent, tempered, angry, and very controlling. None of her close friends and family liked him. He could never let go of Scarlett, and he couldn't stand to see her success at college—a path he didn't take. I'm not even sure if he ever graduated high school.

I yawned and went inside to bed.

Several hours later, the house phone rang. I staggered to the phone, wondering who would be calling in the middle of the night.

It was my best friend's little sister. She said, "Come over … it's Scarlett."

"What?" I asked. A dial tone was the only reply.

I dropped the phone, flustered. I put my shoes on and ran to her house, which was down the street and around the corner. Dawn was breaking, and there was a glow in the cold air. The sun was on the horizon. I ran through the neighborhood park alongside the concrete racquetball courts and quickly came to a halt as police cars surrounded Scarlett's perfectly manicured suburban front lawn.

Her sports car was in the driveway.

A symbol of her success, it was a brand new 1997 Camaro SS, white with orange racing stripes. She was very proud of the gift her parents had given her as a college *signing bonus* for the scholarship she had earned.

I have tons of happy memories at Scarlett's house. Her family welcomed me into their home, and I admired and adored them for that. Scarlett's father was a hardworking man who loved his family. He showed his love by providing for them, and he coached their teams to spend that extra time with them. Scarlett's mom, Lisa, was a stay-at-home mom and always knew what was going on. I don't remember her ever not being there for her family; the girls never came home to an empty house. The house was in order, and she was the boss of it. As teenagers, we were welcome to relax, eat food, or sit around as long as we picked up after ourselves and left the house in the condition we found it in. Sophia, her cute little sister, would pop in and out of the room to see what we were doing. She was all smiles and happy to be in her older sister's presence. They were competitive on and off the field, which made for fun family banter. I often spent the night on their bunk beds and went night swimming with them after we'd finished hitting softballs in their backyard batting cages.

Scarlett set many records as a softball catcher. She was the team captain and fun company. Her physical and mental strength was unparalleled. From a young age, she was groomed and determined to play college ball, and every move she made was in line with this goal. She excelled at both basketball and softball. Down to her core, Scarlett was a phenomenal athlete with blonde hair, blue eyes, and a great physique.

In the late nineties, the majority of full-ride softball scholarships from Arizona State University were awarded to either girls in California or girls who lived out of state. Coach Scott, Scarlett's dad, and Coach Rob created a winning softball program and wanted to keep the girls in state, so they would continue to have the support they needed from parents and the community.

Because of Scarlett's phenomenal ability as catcher, Coach Scott was adamant to keep her in state and turn Arizona State University into a winning program. Scarlett was the first in-state player to receive a full-ride scholarship. Her Storm teammates were soon to follow, and a new trend started.

The driveway looked like a crime scene, and I was baffled as to what could have happened. We were together only a few hours ago. I approached the house slowly, where I found a somber group of authorities. "What happened?" I asked them.

"There was a homicide," the police officer stated.

Scarlett was dead.

Split in two by the pain, it felt like my mind had left my body. Shortly after, the authorities painted a picture of my best friend's death. Scarlett hadn't been murdered—they had ruled her death a suicide. I closed my eyes and imagined her sitting alone in her prized white Camaro with orange racing stripes. She held her dad's gun in her hand in her last moments, and I wondered how alone she had to have felt when she pulled the trigger. The white Camaro with orange racing stripes—once symbolizing a successful future—turned into a painful symbol of death. I always thought she had everything, but that moment showed me there was an entire world of pain that lived underneath the surface of the Scarlett I knew and loved.

Scarlett's death did not make any sense to me—how, what, and why?

Not in any way whatsoever did Scarlett *ever* mention suicide. Though we never talked about suicide, we had shared feelings of rage. We bonded so many times over the rage we both felt, but we were both haunted by different demons. Even when we were hitting a softball as hard as we could, that wasn't enough to release our rage.

I had a car tire in my backyard attached to a pole. The tire had a cut through it, and I used it for batting practice. I would swing a heavy bat through the cut, one hundred swings a day to keep in batting shape. When I returned home the night of Scarlett's death, the sun had risen, and I hit it for hours without batting gloves until my hands were blistered and bloodied.

Numbed by the pain of Scarlett's death without a connection to God, a negative spiral began to brew a perfect storm. The stages of grief were unbearable. I was angry! Why wasn't I with her? Why her and not me? I thought I knew her. She was my god-damned best friend. So many questions ran through my head that I couldn't find the answers to.

This unthinkable event rocked the small town of Glendale—and the club and collegiate softball communities. Although the day of the funeral was bright, a somber mood fell over the day. I looked around and saw tons of people gathered to mourn for the unexpected loss of my best friend. Then, Scarlett's younger sister read the most beautiful poem:

If dreams could build a staircase,
Hers would have no end,
In her ambitions to be a success,
the world became her best friend,
But a sis means more than just a best friend,
especially the kind I've lost,
I'd pay any price to see her once again.
I just wish I knew the cost.
She was the person I wished I could be,
She was wonderful inside and out,
which everyone who knew her could see.
She could light up a room with her smile,
And make everyone else smile, too,
There were endless possibilities to the things she could do.
I know we'll all remember her, and miss her every day,
I wish there were words to make this hurting stop,
but I don't know what to say.
I do know she's looking down on us from heaven up above,
To see that she's the person who we all miss and love.

I LOVE YOU SISTER!!! – Sophia

Everything was a blur for me at the funeral and after. When I woke up two days later, I was still in a fog. Perhaps it was because I had taken a full bottle of pills the night before in the hopes of not waking up. It felt like a bad dream, but it was a new reality. *The pills did not work,* I thought. *I will never have a best friend again. No one will ever accept and share the special moments we shared together. Who will protect me from myself or stop me from hurting others?*

My parents started asking questions instead of demanding I keep to my rigorous practice schedule. "Honey, are you feeling okay?" they would ask. "Is this too much pressure with practice and school?" Wow—what a change. Up until Scarlett's death, my parents had constantly applied the pressure of their expectations onto me, my brother and step-sister to be self-sufficient. They wanted us to be more than *happy kids*. They didn't have money to send me to school, so they needed me to get a scholarship. They viewed playing softball as a ticket to college. Anything short of going all in all the time was frowned upon because I could blow my chance. How different could my life have been if my parents had stayed together—or if we had more money?

My mom was and still is super religious. But the only God I was familiar with was a God of performance. When I performed, my parents loved me. But when I failed, my mother's silence shunned me for days or weeks.

My parents handled me with kid gloves for the remainder of the school year. I returned to college for my sophomore year and finished my last season, but I had no intentions of playing softball ever again. During freshman year, we won the NJCAA National Championship, and during sophomore year, we were runners-up for the National Championship. The sport had left me physically and emotionally broken.

The school provided a support group for students who were affected by suicide. According to the American College Health Association (ACHA), the suicide rate among young adults ages fifteen to twenty-four has tripled since the 1950s, and suicide is currently the second most common cause of death among college students. When I attended the support groups, we shared stories of recognizing or ignoring the signs.

I heard when college students are away from their home, their family, and their friends for the first time, it can lead to suicide. They're living with strangers, far from their support systems. Working under intense pressure with disrupted sleep, eating, and exercise patterns also adds to the chaos. You could hardly design a more stressful situation, particularly when depression or other mental health issues enter the picture.

But this wasn't the case for Scarlett. She was a trailblazer and determined in all she did. I still had no answers as to why her life had to end so soon. As I sat with the support groups and listened with my young ears, I didn't find any comfort. Even though Scarlett was blessed with exceptional athletic talent and was liked by everyone she met, I learned that mental illness has many faces.

There were still so many unanswered questions. Scarlett was survived by her father, mother, and sister. They disagreed with the authorities about the suicide. They launched their own private investigation, which made the whole town talk. Everyone was on eggshells about what to believe. Did her boyfriend kill her? Who else was at the crime scene?

I was unaware of the epidemic of suicide before Scarlett's death. Knowing what I learned in the support group about the signs of suicide, her aggressive behavior could have been a sign. (See Appendix 1) Our behavior was common among many teens in our area. We were very destructive. When the lights went out, there was no telling what would happen. We were like Jekyll and Hyde. By day, we earned good grades and played for winning teams. By night, we roamed the streets, going on sprees of destructive pranks with no regard to who or what we damaged. I knew where my rage came from, but she never mentioned why she raged.

Mailbox baseball was a favorite of ours. All we needed was a truck—sometimes a Chevy or sometimes a Ford—but never an import, a metal bat, and it was *game on*. If the mailbox was knocked loose, we earned a base hit. When we knocked the mailbox completely off, we earned a home run. The one with the lowest points earned the thrill of *lawn jockey*. The lawn jockey was the one who had to jump out of the bed of the navy-blue Chevy truck, go in the front yard to quickly collect lawn ornaments, and jump back in the truck. We traveled only a block or two and then placed the ornaments in another yard. It was our version of ridiculousness.

First, the authorities questioned me. Then, the family's private investigator questioned me months later. Scarlett's blue-collar boyfriend was the last to see her. They had a volatile relationship, and Scarlett's only way to escape him was when she left for college. Christmas break brought them back together and right back into their old patterns, which usually ended in violence. They were so young and restless.

The case finally closed and was once again ruled a suicide.

I buried the memories deep down and went on with my life, but I will always carry a special place in my heart for Scarlett. She will always be the angel on my shoulder.

I will forever be asking *Why her and not me?*

CHAPTER 2

QUIT WISHING YOU HAD SOMEONE ELSE'S LIFE

CHILDHOOD

Nothing happened to you. It's happened for you.
Every disappointment. Every wrong. Every closed
door has helped make you who you are.

—Joel Osteen

In 1992, Glendale, Arizona, located just west of Phoenix, had a small population of 50,000 people. My mom knew the mailman and the check-out lady at the local grocery store, Alpha Beta, where she shopped on Wednesday mornings. To this day, she still talks to everyone she meets. She constantly reminds me, "Strangers are only friends you haven't met yet."

The 1990s were an interesting time in Arizona because cocaine was coming in from Mexico. It was in 1982 when President Ronald Regan declared the war on drugs, and Arizona was a focus point because of the border. This fueled the gang activity. (Today, Glendale Arizona—now five times the population at 250,000—is nationally known as the home of the NFL Cardinals and NHL Coyotes.)

My parents divorced when I was three years old. I didn't have a relationship with my dad after the divorce, and because I was little, I don't remember him living with us before the divorce. Once my daughter Liv was born, we developed a relationship and speak every day now that I am a mother. You know what they say, babies bring people together.

Life was easy growing up as a simple suburban middle-class family. We had one car and a single-family home in a newer suburban development with a carport. My mom, brother, and I went to Sunday school at a small Methodist Church, but at that young age, I did not have a relationship with God. I enjoyed getting dressed for church and playing with the other kids there. Sunday's in our house were recognized as the Sabbath day, which meant no work, no laundry, no lawn mower, and no TV. We went for ice cream after church and sat on the back porch. My mom read the Sunday newspaper, and we played in the back yard. She told stories about despising my father for watching Sunday football and drinking beer. My mom said it was the main reason she could not stay married to him. She prayed the same canned prayer every night at dinnertime. "God is great, God is good, let us thank Him for our food."

I felt connected at home, and I had a happy childhood. My mom told me how blessed I was to have everything I did. I knew I was a cute kid because when my mother and I entered a room, people stopped and smiled. Our beauty warmed the room. Then came the compliments. My mother was a hairdresser, so she loved to dress her hair and mine into extravagant hairstyles. She sewed us matching clothes, and strangers told me I was cute on a regular basis.

As a young child, I remember playing in the cul-de sac with neighborhood kids. Mom constantly said, "Go outside and play. Come in when the streetlight goes on." Wow, how times have changed. I barely let my daughter out of my sight. Life seemed so simple back then.

I was ten years old when I started my period during a school day. Like many other young girls, I thought I was dying! I wondered what the mess was in my pants. Immediately after school, I went to a girl classmate's house and told her and her older sister what happened. My mom and I had not talked about periods or what that meant. They laughed and told me, "It's going to be all right! Here, use this pad. You will be fine. Go home and talk to your mom." I was shocked. *Everyone else is talking to their moms about this except me. Why didn't my mom and I talk about this?*

It served as confirmation for me that my mom didn't accept, I was growing up. I was not her perfect little girl anymore with a cute tan face and hair she could put in ponytails with ringlets. She no longer pictured me as the little girl she could dress up with in matching outfits. Because she wasn't prepared for me getting older, she didn't prepare me for it either. I wished I had the life my friend had with sisters and a mom who understood how important growing up was.

If we didn't talk about it, then she would not face it. On the streets and from cable TV and my friends, I learned about my period, sex, drugs, and alcohol. Our house didn't have any drugs, alcohol or cable TV, but I saw those things while visiting my friend's houses. I saw bottles on the coffee table and smelled something different than cigarettes coming their parent's bathroom. At ten-years-old, I did not know what it was. Now, marijuana is legal in some states.

It was the first week of seventh grade, which was the super awkward time when everyone's hormones were changing. Junior high was difficult, in part because of the way the zoning worked. Three schools merged together for two years. Who came up with that idea? Let's put all the hormonal teenagers together to prey on each other. It was like walking onto a battlefield every day. My best friend Karina and I stuck very close together. She was mixed-race, part Pacific Islander. She never knew her dad. He was in the service and met her mom while he was stationed in Hawaii. She also had a stepdad. We'd daydream like Nancy Drew and talk about how we would find our dads. They would be so happy to see us and would welcome us with open arms, followed by, *no one will hurt my baby girl, I got you.* What a dream that was.

We were both very tall and with our other similarities, we always had each other's backs. Immediately, we received unwanted attention from the eighth-grade boys, which turned the eighth-grade girls against us right away. Our bodies were growing and shaping. My little-girl cuteness turned into young-woman attractiveness. It caused cat calls and verbal taunts, which made the girls hate us and shout bad words at us. School was no longer a fun, worry-free zone. We were like *babes in the wood.*

My friend and her brother planned to attend a back-to-school get-together. I thought I should go and try to make new friends. My friend's brother was in high school, and we were in junior high. I went home first to check-in, then headed over. My girl-friend never showed up. Back then, we didn't have cell phones or pagers to stay connected. When I got to the house party there were no adults home, only a mix of teenagers I had never seen before. They were smoking and rolling blunts. My friend's brother handed me a cup, and I held on to it for dear life. The entire situation felt wrong, but I still sat there—a stranger among all those older kids, holding a strange drink in my hands.

My friend's brother said, "Come with me."

I thought he was going to ask me to leave, but he led me to a back room. The hair on the back of my neck stood up. I asked what we were doing and where we were going. I asked if Karina was there. He pushed his body on to me and I pushed back, but he was a lot bigger than me. My drink flung out of my hand, and he forced himself on me. He was sexually assaulting me, but I didn't know how to stop him. I struggled silently until I went limp. It was like my mind had left my body, and I was in shock. Split in two by the pain, my body trembled all over. He said, "Don't worry, I won't tell my sister. Pull yourself together, and then you should leave."

After a few minutes I stopped crying, put my clothes back on and walked out of the bedroom to the hall. I quietly exited the house. I ran home, but no one was home when I got there.

Lonely and scared, I took a shower and went to bed. I wished and hoped it had been a bad dream.

I returned to the junior high the following Monday. I thought if I never spoke of it then it never happened.

It only took a day or two until the rumors spread that I was sexually active. My friend's brother had bragged about the *encounter* as though it was two-sided and not an assault. When my brother heard about it, he told my parents. My mom remarried when I was 10 years old. She was so mad at me she didn't speak to me for at least a week. I had no one to tell what had really happened. They had already labeled me, and after that, I was never the same. My emotional wall went up, preventing anyone from the truth of what had really happened at that party. Guarded and filled with internal rage, I got into several fights on and off campus with girls who harassed me. When I got suspended, either in-school or out-of-school, it was a relief. At least I didn't have to worry that day.

After that, my best girlfriend was mad at me because she thought I liked her brother. She didn't really know that I didn't like him—I wanted to kill him. I constantly plotted in my head of ways to poison him. I didn't have enough guts to shoot him, although it did cross my mind. My world crashed as my best friendship was splintered. I got in a fight at an away game on the basketball court and established a reputation as a fighter. I was disconnected from my friends, my brother wouldn't even look at me, and my parents were disgusted and disappointed. And this was all because I was at the wrong place at the wrong time. My relationship with my mom never recovered. That was when I realized she didn't care about my feelings, only about my reputation. I realized my search for a protector would last forever.

HIGH SCHOOL

Yelling, storming out, and slamming doors was typical at home. My stepdad and I spent a lot of time together and got along great for several years. He even coached me in softball, but in high school, we repelled each other like oil and water. He and my mom set boundaries for me—a *tough-love* kind of jail. But I broke them and was a constant disappointment. My mom made it known she did not like my choices. She shared her racism when she told me not to hang out with *those* kids, or I would be judged. She asked if I wanted to end up pregnant or in jail like them. *They are my only friends,* I thought. *If that's how she feels, why don't we move north like everyone else, to where my club softball friends live? Then, I could go to a predominately white school.* In my neighborhood, I was becoming a minority and friendship with everyone was a survival skill, and I didn't know any different.

One time, I stood face to face with my stepdad and told him to get out of my way. My mom's fist reached over and punched me in the face. I was ballistic and stunned and realized I had no one to trust. My jaw dropped when she called the cops and said I was unruly. Whose parents call the cops on their kids? I had not heard of such a thing. When the authorities arrived, I pleaded with the cops to please take me with them. In retrospect, I think white privilege was why they didn't want to take me with them because they wanted to keep me out of the system. After all, my mom had drilled in me for so long that *those kids* always ended up pregnant or in jail. Maybe they thought that, too. I didn't want to be there anymore, and my parents did not want me there either.

I was no longer my mom's little girl. She had turned her back on me, moved on, and gotten married. It was not my fault I grew into a teenager. She was in love with the idea of having a young daughter, not a teenager or independent daughter. Her emotional intelligence couldn't handle the real-world daily problems and obstacles a teenager goes through. I didn't feel safe in my home any longer, and that was unsettling. The softball field was the only place I ever felt like I belonged as a teenager. Everywhere else I went, I tried, usually unsuccessfully, to fit in.

The cops didn't take me that night, to my surprise. So, I packed a garbage bag full of clothes and left. No one came after me. I stayed down the street with a friend. There were four kids in the family, so one more was no bother. They had a pool and a third car (it was my perception that they were rich). Their mom was friends with her kids, took them shopping, and talked about boys with them. There was no talk about boys at my house. It was more like a convent. After all, my mother's mindset was *If we don't talk about it, it's not happening*. I think I probably over explain everything now that I have a daughter because I want her to hear it from me.

My high school seemed to be an equal mix of three races: white, black, and Hispanic. The neighborhoods were divided accordingly. The shady liquor stores, pawn shops, and tattoo parlors were a few miles south. The corner became very familiar to me, even a routine stop. It was on that corner where the Bloods and Crips collided at night. Anyone brave enough could buy or sell drugs, contraband, firearms, etc. I was sure to get there before 10:00 p.m. because illegal things happened there after that. I purchased alcohol underage, which became my social currency. My presence in the liquor store was always welcomed. I felt safe there, no matter how dangerous that corner was.

The upperclassmen boys started to notice me, but I didn't want anything to do with them. I thought if I partnered with one of the tallest, biggest, *baddest* football players—he would be my protector. I was right. For two years, I *belonged* to a football player who was in a gang—his name was tattooed on my ring finger. Boys my age were petrified to talk to me. There were rumors that he hurt some of my classmates if he thought they liked me. I saw him when it was convenient for him. He was mostly on the streets on the weekends, so the relationship didn't take up much of my time. It was more of a label, a status symbol. He was good at football and had hopes and dreams of pursuing it professionally, but the streets took him like the scene from *Boys In the Hood*.

It was sunset on a Friday night. We hung out early before then went out on the streets. That evening they left in a stolen car and off they went to take care of *business*. He visited me at the end of the night and tapped on my bedroom window. When I opened the window, he was trembling, his skin white as a ghost. I had seen this tremble a few times before, but not to this extreme. We jumped my wooded planked backyard fence and sat in the bottom of an empty swimming pool of the abandoned house behind mine. We shared a cigarette, and he told me about his night. This night though, he was a little different. He said he might have to leave for a while. He was sweaty, pale, and unsteady even as we sat there. I said, "Okay, I'll see you when you get back." I didn't want to know what had happened, but the hair on the back of my neck told me it was a horrific situation. We embraced, and that was the last time I saw him.

The next day, I heard about a drive-by shooting a few blocks from my house that night—a gang altercation. A civilian was murdered in the crossfire, and my boyfriend was picked up for murder (or accessory to murder, not sure which). He went to jail, and I never heard from him again.

Suddenly, that twinge in my stomach was gone—I was mentally and physically set free. My mom didn't hesitate when I told her I wanted to remove the tattoo. I had the tattoo burned off my finger with a laser at the doctor's office. The worst smell ever is human skin burning, but it was the smell of my freedom. Don't deny your inner voice because it is your sixth sense telling you something isn't quite right.

You know what they say—idle times are the devil's workshop. It's best to join a team and stay out of trouble. High School and club sports teams were a big part of my life and a one-way ticket to my dream of *getting the hell out of this small town*. In high school, I played varsity softball at fourteen years old. My talent placed me with the sixteen, seventeen, and eighteen-year old's. Can you imagine how insecure I was? I was a part of the winning season and started every game that year at first base. We won state runner-up. My parents were so happy I was playing, they didn't question anything I was doing or anyone I was socializing with. The girls were my teammates, and as long as I had good grades and was playing well, I pretty much could—and did—run wild. Alcohol eased my insecurities about fitting in with the older girls.

I had the gift (or the curse) of morphing into whatever person I needed to be in whatever situation I was in. Tall, blonde, and tan, with a smile and air of confidence that said I belonged exactly where I was. I made myself appear older than fourteen, which put me in some sticky and violent situations. I cultivated the skill of lying at an early age and had no qualms about it. It was a survival skill I needed to exist. My side hustle was over-charging underage students for alcohol. If they drove, I bought the alcohol for a small fee. I had the confidence to walk into a middle eastern family-run liquor store. The store smelled of old cardboard and dust. The owner handed me the large order with an extra small bottle only for me. He winked and said, "See you next week." When I glanced over and saw a gun on the bottom of the back shelf, it gave me a feeling of security: *Oh good, they're armed, just in case anything happens.* What the heck was I thinking, and why did this not trigger danger to me? Instead, I was drawn to it. The florescent light flickered, and I walked out with my arms full of the night's spirits. These stores were scary for most but for me. I felt the rush of the ask and the receive. I don't recall ever being turned away.

When I walked the halls of the high school the day after our state championship, it was an out of body experience because of the triumph afterward. I remember the excitement of getting ready for the party, the rush of getting the alcohol, and then celebrating with the softball team all night before the blackout.

After we won state runner-up, we celebrated with a house party. The background music of Biggie Smalls and Tupac filled the air. Plastic cups with Mad Dog 20/20 and Boone's Farm were everywhere. Marijuana circulated around the house, and there was a supply of menthol cigarettes, too. I sat back and enjoyed the buzz. Suddenly, the night went black, like someone had pulled the curtains shut. I was fourteen years old when I experienced my first blackout.

The next day, I tried to piece together the night before. At the time, we didn't have cell phones or video recordings to get a true depiction. Throughout the day, I received different versions of what happened from different people who were there.

The young age of fourteen was the beginning of a blank space. Like Rachael, played by Emily Blunt in the movie, *Girl on the Train*, I was never quite sure of what I took part in or witnessed in the state of black out. This left a blackhole in my soul that I continued to fill with alcohol and other substances.

Am I lying about what happened that night if I was in a black out? I wondered. When I heard about the events, I felt cloudy. I listened and said, "Not sure," or "Yeah," but deep down, I didn't know. My life with trap doors continued.

THE HIGH SCHOOL GRADUATION LIMO RIDE

The stretch limo arrived, and it was beautiful, long, and white. Glancing back at my modest childhood home, I realized it would never look the same now that I was on my way to adulting. I said goodbye to my parents with big hugs. They stood in the carport and waved. I was going to see them at the venue in a few hours for the high school graduation ceremony. They were so proud (and relieved) they had gotten me through this stage of life. I knew my mom and stepdad raised me to graduate high school and go to college. I could sense their relief they had completed that stage of parenting and were counting the days until I left. I was the youngest and the last one out.

I was the first on my mom's side of the family to go to college—with an athletic scholarship. The high school graduation was my last event with friends from the *hood*. In the fall, I planned to attend college and enter the world as an adult.

The summer air was warm, and the sun was shining. It was a hot May day in Arizona. We had planned several stops to pick up five of my classmates. The giddiness of my friends was hard to contain. We were so happy, and we celebrated with drinks in the car. We took pictures with our disposable cameras at all our families' homes.

With ruby red caps and gowns adorned, we arrived at the venue an hour and a half later.

We exited the car like a scene from the movie *The Hangover*. The hot wind blew our hair. We were so proud to wear our beautiful, classy graduation dresses. As the hot summer breeze continued and triumphant music played in our heads, we knew high school was over finally.

The venue was massive, ornate, and sophisticated. There was a pleasant rumble as families gathered. Elation was in the air.

Before the ceremony, while we were putting on our caps and gowns in the green room, my female principal—a dead ringer for Jane Lynch from *Glee*—approached me to help pin on my hat. She kept saying how proud she was of me, and she said I would be called up and recognized three times. This was uncommon, because statistically, the chance of graduating at my high school was only 85%. An even smaller percentage of students went to college, so graduating was not a given at my high school. Teenage pregnancies, jail, or dropouts were not unheard of by any means. In the 1996 graduation program, I was recognized for graduating with my class, for my GPA, and for a female athletic scholarship.

"Let me help you with that," Mrs. Principal said and continued to praise me for bringing so many accolades to the school and giving girls hope everywhere.

"What is that smell?" she asked as she pinned on my graduation hat with a bobby pin.

She bent closer to me and sniffed. "Have you been drinking?" she demanded to know.

"Yes, in the car on the way," I said without missing a beat. "We were celebrating!"

"You cannot walk if you've been drinking," *Jane* said sternly.

I paused for a moment.

"No worries," I replied. "I'll head back to the limo." I removed my cap and gown, gathered some friends and attendees, and continued the party in the car.

The ceremony began without me.

My best friend walked by my parents and told them, "Crystal cannot walk."

Their first thought was to wonder if I broke my leg or something. The ceremony continued, a milestone I missed because of my *affliction*. My name was called—nothing but crickets.

To this day, I am reminded of the legacy I left at the high school. Every year during the senior meeting, the class reviewed the top five rules: *No matter who you are, you will not walk if you are any degree intoxicated. It continues,...not even if you have a scholarship and are to be called up three times...We have a zero-tolerance policy.*

CHAPTER 3
QUIT TAKING THE EDGE OFF

MARTINIS AND MOTHERHOOD

The thunderbolt of waking up to discover
a blank space where pivotal scenes should be.
My evenings come with trap doors.

—Sarah Hepola, *Black Out*

My twentieth birthday was a great reason to black out my feelings. I was with teammates and several financial donors of the state university sports program. We danced to the local cover band and drank all night, feeling no pain or responsibility. It was another epic, meaningless night. When the night came to an end, the girls and I piled into a car and headed back to campus. We had been laughing and giggling on stage with the band. We shook the tambourine to "Brown Eyed Girl" by Van Morrison as we talked over each other about the night. Another alcohol-fueled, legendary night was behind us, and we'd gotten away with it. Less than five minutes into the drive on Scottsdale Road, the red and blue lights flickered in the review mirror. The echo of the siren startled me. I pulled over thinking it couldn't be for me and they would pass by. As I pulled off to the right, the lights followed me. I was pulled over by Scottsdale finest PD fresh out of the academy, eager to prove themselves and unwilling to bend any rules.

"Step out of the car." We looked at each other and giggled. "Where are you headed?" he demanded.

"We have practice in the morning and are going back to campus," I explained. "We're college athletes."

He then asked the passenger to get out of the car, "Blow in this." He paused. "I hope you girls had fun, but none of you can drive. Call someone to drive you home." We called our assistant coach to pick us up and drive the car back to campus—none of us dared to call our parents.

That night was two months after Scarlett's suicide death. I was out of my mind, numbing the pain. It was 1998 before the DUI laws were not so strict. I went to court and pled *no contest.* I was assigned an *underage consumption ticket.* It resulted in a one-game suspension, a monetary fine, and five mandatory Alcoholics Anonymous classes, also known as meetings. The meetings planted the seed of realization that my drinking was different than others'. I took the test they handed you in the meetings and was relieved that it was not a test I wanted to pass. It was a test about drinking habits—no studying required. (Appendix II) Alcoholism is the only self-diagnosed disease.

My mom and stepdad attended the following preseason scrimmage game but found me on the bench. Once again, they thought I was hurt since I had not started. They later found out it was due to alcoholic-related consequences. My parents took the tough-love approach—I received the silent treatment until enough time passed. When the silent treatment was over, we picked up where we left off. They never addressed it.

STILL BORN – ANGEL WALLEN

We won a national championship my freshman year in college. My sophomore year was all fucked up. Scarlett died, and the head coach was crossing the line with a player. I was not sure what was going on, but I heard rumors. He was definitely not a protector. We were not supposed to work off-campus as a rule of our scholarships. However, I took a job at a local sports bar in town on Thursday, Friday, and Saturday nights, which meant I stopped socializing with the team on the weekends. I served the alcohol so I would not drink it, which saved me quite a bit of money. As one of the few who didn't receive an allowance from their parents, my parents made it very clear I would have to pay my own way once I was out of the house. I made up to $100 a weekend on tips and saved it all. When sophomore year ended, I really didn't want to play ball anymore. The sport I used to love brought me emotional and physical pain. When I thought of the sport, it reminded me of my aching back and losing my best friend. I wanted to go to the university as a regular student, not travel in a pack of thirteen girls with a male coach whom I didn't trust anymore. That was when I decided to quit playing softball.

In the fall, I rented a room and attended ASU. I dropped twenty pounds because I no longer had to over-train with the team and eat cafeteria food. I was feeling fantastic. It was springtime, and I was excited to see a fling whose company I really enjoyed. He was only in town for a short three months for spring training each year. It was easy, glamorous, and exciting. We spent the last two springs together during his stay for spring training in January, February, and March. If we went out, it was usually with a group of three guys. I was his girl, and the others would pick up random girls. He had a driver, and we were escorted to the back door of the club and directly to the VIP section, where bottles were served. I enjoyed the night out with all the pretty people. He made me feel safe.

I was never really into guys my age, preferring guys a few years older and wiser. Many had told me I was an old soul. I socialized mostly with people out of college who had lifestyles I wanted. There was nobody else—my spring fling had my heart—and I thought there was a chance we would end up together.

For two years, we had a seasonal relationship. I was enamored with him. Nobody could stand up to him. I thought he could be the one if the timing was right. Our relationship was seasonal—I didn't want to go on the road with him. I didn't want that lifestyle. Free from the obligation of a team, I was living on my own. We were the perfect couple who laughed a lot and were very relaxed together. He had been playing Major League Baseball for several years and was on his way to setting new hitting records. It was a magical time. I stayed with him at his leased mansion where we hung out and chilled on nights when we weren't out on the town. He took everything he did seriously, whether it was work or relaxation. We had great chemistry, and we had a lot in common. When the season started, he left to do what he did best, play baseball. The months passed by so quickly.

I had heard he was married and getting divorced, but he denied it, and I wanted to believe him. How could he be married when we were so good together? But whether he was married or not, I knew I was not the only woman in his life. He was a young, rich, attractive professional athlete. It was no surprise to me that he had women in every town. But I believed we were meant to be, and I would outlast all the others. Even though I only saw him for three months a year, our relationship wasn't *temporary*. When he left town, I knew he'd be back the next year. I knew he'd come back to me. The relationship was like a fairy tale for me, despite how unconventional it was. I thought he was *it,* the one.

I ignored the other women in his life because he treated me with kindness, and I felt safe with him. I also ignored the needles laying all over the mansion. The team had a very strict steroid regimen. I saw all the guys inject in the morning and at night. Steroid laws were different back then—there *were* laws, but they weren't as strict. When the old stuff was outlawed, the latest doctor developed new stuff, and the athletes would use that. It wasn't only steroids, either—whenever I went over, there was cocaine, alcohol, and other drugs. I had been around drugs and alcohol in high school and college, so I didn't even bat an eye because I was under the impression everyone was doing it.

The summer approached, and to my surprise, I was pregnant. *Oh shit, what now?* I had just lost Scarlett, divorced my sport, and now I was going to create a new life. I didn't want to cause any fuss or be needy, so I didn't call him right away. There were no delusions about our relationship—it was one of convenience, and it was seasonal. By the time I visited the doctor, I was six months pregnant.

I went home to tell my parents. Because I had encountered their lack of emotion on previous occasions, the disappointment on my mom's face was oh too familiar and recognizable.

She said, "I will not raise your baby," and nothing else was said about it.

I left with a sense of clarity. From the time I turned thirteen, I had always felt like I was on my own. As an adult, I was still on my own. *I will survive this,* I thought. *I will have the baby and then call him.* Having the baby was my priority, and I would figure out later how to handle the rest of it. I quickly visited my guidance counselor and said, "I need to graduate as soon as possible." We looked at all the credits I had accumulated over the last three years. She said I could graduate with a BA Communications Degree, but I still needed three more classes, two of which I could take online. I had done something right—my diploma was in sight. After some time had passed, my parents called and said, "Come home. You can live here until you figure out what to do."

So, I returned home and started saving money. I did what I knew best and worked at a local country bar on Thursday, Friday, and Saturday nights. There was live bull-riding and live country music. I didn't have any trouble getting jobs. No one knew I was pregnant except my parents and my stepsister. No one knew I was pregnant except my parents and my stepsister. My belly grew, but I was thin and didn't have as big a bump as some women did. It also helped that my breasts were growing along with my belly—I could throw on a loose top and you'd never know I was pregnant.

I transferred from campus to a closer satellite campus of ASU on the west side of town, studying all day, resting at night, and working on the weekends. My social life consisted of serving Bud Lights for $2.25 and receiving a seventy-five-cent tip for each beer. I felt safe there like I belonged—I stayed in my lane, collected money, and got out. The bouncers kept a close eye on me, and no one really bothered me. One of the bouncers had a crush on me. He resembled Garth Brooks. He was nice and kind and big and burley from the mid-west. He was over six feet tall, handsome, and wore a black t-shirt with a straw cowboy hat. All the girls liked him, and he liked me. He asked me out every week to hang out or to have a beer. I kindly declined, week after week, and said I had to study.

It was October, and the air was getting a chill at night. The State Fair was in town. He asked me to the fair. I considered going, for this might be the last time I could attend the fair without a child. So, I said, "Sure, why not?" I explained I didn't like rides, which was a lie, but it was a way to still conceal my baby bump. He had a kind face and was a family guy. The kind you would want to raise a family in the country with. He picked me up that night in his lifted pick-up truck. I felt like such an imposter. *What a nice guy I am leading on,* I scolded myself. *If only he knew.*

We arrived at the State Fair with slot machines dinging, carnies yelling, and the smell of funnel cake filling the air. A normal twenty-year-old would be in heaven, but not me. I had something growing inside. I could not help staring at every baby I saw. After we had walked around for several hours, I started to lose my balance and started cramping. I was an expert at excuses, so he was not alarmed at all when I said I had to go home. Even though I was in extreme pain, I was quick at covering it up. The night came to an end.

He drove me home around 10:00 p.m. since I had school in the morning. He walked me to the house back gate through the carport, said good night, and kissed my face. I couldn't enjoy it because my uterus was exploding. After quickly saying good night, I thanked him and told him I'd see him tomorrow night at work. I would *not* see him the next night, though—I was about to give birth.

I staggered to the bathroom in pain, holding onto the walls of the hallway. After making it to the toilet, I pulled my pants down, and what felt like a tsunami rushed out of me. There was blood everywhere. I screamed for my mom, and she hurried in franticly and saw the blood. "Your water broke!" she exclaimed. "Hurry, let's go!"

What? I couldn't believe it. *I am early in the third trimester! Maybe I have my date wrong. Afterall,* I hadn't gotten any prenatal care besides a prenatal vitamin, and I had only known about my pregnancy for three months. So, yes, *maybe* I had my date wrong. My mom pulled up my pants and helped me walk to the Ford Silverado in the driveway. My stepdad got in and drove us to the emergency room.

The fluorescent lights glared, and the staff rushed me inside the emergency room in a wheelchair screaming and aching, my pants a liquid bloody mess. They threw me up on a table and the nurse said, "This baby is coming *now*." I was in excruciating pain, and I was unprepared for that because I hadn't taken any birthing classes. I thought, *I am not ready for this.*

The baby was stillborn. I was numb and barely blinked—the experience was unreal. The hospital wrapped her up in blanket, put a cap on her head, and went through the process of foot-printing her. I received a death certificate with the name I had given her on it—Angel Wallen. She was cremated and placed in a plot at the Methodist Church I grew up in.

As a young teenager, I thought I would marry a baseball player. I played softball and all my friends were athletes, so it made sense. When I started dating a professional baseball player who was at the top of his game and in perfect physical shape, it felt like that dream was coming true. We were both healthy, good-looking athletes. So, when I got pregnant with his child, a small part of me thought it was Scarlett—athletic, beautiful Scarlett—coming back to me. I thought if it was a girl, I would name her Scarlett.

Stillborn. How could this have happened? We were both so healthy. Well, I wasn't actually healthy—I didn't receive any prenatal care. I hadn't known I was pregnant for six months, so I kept drinking that whole time. I stopped when I found out, but I guess it was too late. I ignored the needles I saw at the rented mansion and believed the excuses I heard about vitamins. He later admitted to the grand jury that he'd been using steroids after setting some homerun records on his east coast team. I never spoke to him again. Our romance died with our baby.

I went home that night and slept for at least two days. I was unable to look at my parents because I didn't want to see that sense of relief on their faces. I didn't return to the country bar or the handsome country bouncer. After receiving another chance at life and love, I didn't want it. I walked around in a shell of my body—emotionally spent from the loss of my best friend and my stillborn baby. After taking way too many pills, I fell asleep, hoping not to wake up. But again, my suicide attempt failed.

When I woke up, I reached under my shirt to feel my stomach—it was flat and tender. Wow the baby is gone and I am alive. A week later or so my immediate family and I had a small ceremony for the baby at the church. I did what I did best and reinvented myself with weight loss and blonder hair, and I moved on. Graduation was coming up, and I was done dating athletes. I planned to look for a life partner—a protector who held power and not fame. After my relationship with the baseball player ended, I decided not to date athletes anymore—I wouldn't even socialize with them. I couldn't deal with the lifestyle because I was jaded, and I knew I wanted stability. Who I associated with needed to change, so I got new friends. I wanted to start a business and use my diploma as my ticket to a new life. For whatever reason, God gave me another chance to do it right. I traded in the jersey for the suit, still in search of a protector.

LOVE AT FIRST SIGHT

It was love at first sight. I graduated from Arizona State University in December, a semester early, because I thought I was baby bound. Now, free to start over, I wanted to travel. With my degree in hand, I was on the move seeking employment in Las Vegas, Los Angeles, and New York. My family was rooted in Arizona, but I yearned for a different experience. After all, there were so many people in the world and places to see. In December of 2001, the week I graduated, my friends were on break from college for the holidays. I was traveling with a group of my softball friends and their parents to Las Vegas. The group was going for a vacation, but I was looking for my first real job out of college. I had been there for three days, and my last interview was at The Venetian hotel in Vegas. During my meeting, Michael walked in the room, and my interviewer got up to meet him at the door. We locked eyes, and he left. When the interview was over, I was asked to join them for dinner. He mentioned we were both from Arizona. The crew I was traveling with left earlier that day. I packed my bag and was walking through the hotel lobby when I ran into Michael again, and we locked eyes again. He approached me and asked, "Aren't you joining us for dinner?"

"I am heading to the airport," I responded. "I have been here three days. I am packed and checked out."

He said, "Take a later flight, and join us for dinner at Nine Steak House. Put your bag at the bell desk. Chris mentioned we were both from Arizona and that we were both single. Let's go for a drink until dinner time, and you can catch a later flight." So, I went with Michael for a drink and dinner.

We shared a similar story that was related to 9/11. When the tragedy struck the USA, it was human nature to check on all the ones you loved. We both knew after 9/11 that the relationships we were in at the time were not lifelong.

His blue eyes were warm, and he had a kind demeanor. Could this be my prince charming in a blazer with a crisp white-collar shirt, a suit jacket, and jeans? He had the James Bond look and reminded me of Pierce Brosnan in the movie, *The Thomas Crown Affair* (A favorite movie of mine).

We went for a drink at the V Bar in The Venetian hotel, and our chemistry was undeniable.

Then, we had dinner at the Nine Steak House at Palms hotel. There was a group of twelve or so, but he and I chatted with each other like no one else was in the room.

It was 10:00 p.m., and I had to leave the strip to catch the last flight back to Phoenix. He asked me to stay and fly out with him in the morning.

I considered it. "Well, we can if we stay up all night and take the 5:30 a.m. flight back." I suggested. He agreed, and the magical night continued. He had many clients in Vegas and took me to all the hot spots where they knew him by name. We were so interested in each other, and the conversation flowed like it never had before in my life.

The night had turned to morning. It seemed like no time had passed at all, like the world stood still, and it was just us. All the other people were simply extras in our movie. We went back to The Venetian to pick up my suitcase from the bell stand and his laptop brief case from his room. He opened the doors to his hotel room, and voilà—it was the largest hotel room I had ever seen. After he grabbed his laptop, we headed for the airport.

The sun rose as we landed in Phoenix. I was living in a studio apartment by myself in downtown Phoenix. He declined dropping me off and drove to his house instead. He said he had an international call, didn't want to be late, and preferred calling from home.

I laid on the couch and watched him walk around the pool on a phone call. He was a great guy, and I was at peace. I dozed off on the couch, and I woke up hours later. He drove me back to my place, but it would be the last time. The next time I went to see him for a visit, I never left. He had two boys, ages two and four at the time. They were with him every other weekend. I witnessed first-hand what an amazing dad he was. I had met my life partner, and I was in love. We lovingly talked about having a baby girl together.

STAY ON THE MAT

It was a hot summer day in Arizona. I was lounging poolside at a local, popular resort with friends, day drinking, and soaking in the sun. Steve, my long-time gay friend, was getting antsy because there was no one there he was attracted to. After a few hours and a great tan later, he said he was going to yoga, and I should join him.

"I don't know what yoga is, but it sounds relaxing," I agreed without too much thought. I was up for anything new in my vodka-altered state. We wrapped ourselves in sarongs, slipped on our flip-flops, and headed to old town for a yoga class. When we walked in, we received a very warm welcome.

The svelte studio owner came over to greet us and said, "Welcome! So, you're a first-time student? Take it easy and stay on the mat." She looked me up and down. I didn't know what yoga was at the time, but she looked like a yoga ninja because her aura was different than anything I had experienced before.

We entered the room, and I gasped. It was hot, dark, and quiet. Steve laid out our rented mats and towels. The mats were placed down, then a towel covered the mat. There were two straight rows with the mats about twelve inches apart. Steve smiled and placed a cold-water bottle above my mat. We sat on the mats and made small talk in the dark. Then the lights turned on.

Wow, that's bright. I felt stunned and took a drink of water.

The yoga instructor walked in the room and shut the door behind her. She had a slender build, sleek black hair, and cute black small shorts. After she introduced herself, she began the class. She instructed us to do deep breathing and to stand with our hands clasped under our chins. Beads of sweat began to roll down the middle of my back. She reminded us to stay on the mat and focus on ourselves.

Stay on the mat. She had already said that. *Why is she telling the whole class? How hard can it be to stay on the mat?* I thought to myself.

The loud breathing of the people around the class was awkward, exhaling through the mouth like a lion. Wow. She called out, "Half-moon! Stand in the middle of your mat. Feet together nicely, clasp your hands over your head, lock your elbows. No bend in the elbows! Focus one point in the mirror, and focus on your third eye. Hips forward, lengthen the spine up to the ceiling. Now, bend to the right and left, warming up both sides of the body."

I was in the front row, so I glanced in the mirror to look around the room. Everyone was making a curve with their body. I pushed my hips to the left side harder, locked my elbow tighter, clasped my hands tightly together, and quickly focused back on myself.

"Right and left, right and left," the instructor continued. "When you cannot stretch anymore, stop in the middle—hips forward, elbow locked—now bend to the right side, and hold it."

My knees started crying, and sweat was pouring out of my body. *What is this?*

"Mouth closed, breathe in and out. Chin up, stretch to the corner of the room, push your hips to the left beyond your flexibility."

I kept holding the pose. *This is the longest sixty seconds, ever.* My face started to fade in and out as I tried to focus on my reflection in the mirror. I felt my body begin to wobble, and my vision became blurry. No longer able to focus on my reflection, my face was fading from view. I blinked my eyes quickly to refocus and everything went black.

When I woke up in the lobby of the studio, I saw a team of firemen standing over me. My eyelids flickered, my body was wet, and I felt cold. I was lying on the hard floor dressed only in a yoga outfit. The instructor talked to the firemen, and my vision came back.

"What happened?" I asked, blinking my eyes to refocus. Embarrassed, I had no idea how powerful yoga was with the combination of breath and movement in a sequential series to heal the body from the inside out. The fact is it opens you up to release the poison and bad energy out. Wow, I realized I could not stand in a yoga room for ten minutes. From the outside, I looked like a perfect specimen—toned, lean, tan—but what was going on inside of me?

I was sweating vodka and tasted salt in my mouth.

"You passed out," the handsome fireman said as he put his hand out to help me sit me up. "We are going to take you to the hospital to check you out and give you more fluids."

I snapped to attention, flustered, and shouted, "No! I cannot go to the hospital. I am fine." I looked to Steve, and he grinned. Already embarrassed enough, going to the hospital would just add insult to injury. Besides, I didn't want my husband to know what had happened. The studio owner glared at Steve and said, "Take her home."

The fireman handed me a piece of paper to sign on the *refuse to go to the hospital* line. I scribbled on it and looked at my friend and said, "Take me home."

After a few days of processing another botched life episode, the phrase *Just stay on your mat* kept replaying in my head. A week later when I went back to the same studio to try yoga again. The owner welcomed me back and said, "It's not your fault. What was Steve thinking, bringing you in here drunk?"

JUST STAY ON YOUR MAT

Drunk? I pondered.

This time, I did not push myself too hard. I was not *day drinking*—instead, I caught the natural high that exercise produces. I made it; I did it. I stayed on my mat for ninety minutes. I was like a little girl, jumping up and down inside. I was hooked. After that day, I was a dedicated student for several years before I became a teacher myself. Because of my first yoga experience, I have so much empathy for new students.

I am not flexible are the most common words I hear when I prescribe yoga to a client as their personal trainer. I remind them, "Flexibility starts in the mind. Just stay in the room on the mat, and take it easy."

You never really know what anyone is going through when they walk in the door of a yoga studio. A normal person walks into their first class and defends their practice before they've even started. They say things like, "Oh, I have not worked out in so long. I am out of shape." I remind them not to push and lay down as much as needed. That way they can stay on the mat and in the room for the entire ninety minutes.

I just smiled and thought, *If you only knew what happened my first class.*

TRYING TO GET PREGNANT

I had the RIDs: restless, irritable, and discontent. The feeling continued in a vicious way. I was ready to settle into marriage and get off the weekend binging cycle. We had the boys every other weekend. When we didn't, we enjoyed each other's company with bottles of wine, martinis, and a passion. When the weekend was over, Michael would go back to work leaving me feeling empty and anxious. *A baby will fix my loneliness*, I thought, so we tried to get pregnant. We agreed we both wanted a baby girl.

No luck after a year.

We sought the counsel of a fertility doctor. Boy, was he strange! He seemed like a modern-day God with all his mysterious, modern fertility interventions. We tried artificial insemination a couple of times, but I never liked the idea of IVF, the trend of designer babies, or interfering with the natural process. I decided to change everything.

I looked into a yoga college, desperately wanting to stop my routine of binge drinking and surround myself with healthy, like-minded people. Determined to prime my body for a baby, I considered yoga teacher training programs and chose the certification that was the most rigorous. It was a hot yoga certification program set for the following fall semester. The contract said, "No drinking," so the plan was perfect. If I changed my environment, the cravings would stop. It was my most dramatic approach to put the cork in the bottle.

Next, I called a family meeting to let them know I would be out of the country for nine weeks, and I wasn't sure how much communication I'd have with them. I also told them everything was all right. They pulled me aside and asked if I was going to rehab, to which I said no and laughed it off. It was my attempt to heal myself.

This nine-week training was in Acapulco, Mexico. I was with three hundred people who spoke seven different languages. It was my way to start fresh, meet new people who were unaware of my blackouts, study, and work hard. The nine-week course was anything but easy. It was very stressful and controversial, and it was also physically and emotionally draining day and night—everything but relaxing. We were hungry, sleep-deprived, and some would say brain-washed. This was a familiar environment, though, because of my college softball training. After a few weeks of living at the Princess hotel on the beaches of Acapulco, I soon found my drinking buddies. So much for changing my environment.

I rationalized my weekend drinks—there was controversy and conflict within the administration of the yoga organization I had joined. It was stressful to be around and spending the weekend poolside at another hotel with a coconut cocktail seemed to be the solution.

The drinking-related blackouts continued.

When I completed the nine weeks of rigorous yoga training, I felt emotionally strong. Cut off from reality of what was happening in the US economy, I had big dreams again. I restored my faith in myself, and I had plans to return home, have a baby, and open my own yoga studio. The economy took a downturn, though, and I became a teacher instead of an owner.

OUR LITTLE GIRL

I thought my drinking problem had dissipated. We had a healthy baby girl. When I got pregnant, I was able to stop drinking and enjoy the occasional glass of red wine at dinner parties. After being married for several years and co-raising my two stepsons, I was elated to be pregnant. I believed a baby would force me to grow up and be responsible for someone else. I would have no choice but to be self-less.

Because I breastfed for over a year, I kept the alcohol away. When I stopped breast feeding, the binge drinking started again with a vengeance. I realized drinking after pregnancy was never the same. I was constantly trying to recreate the fun of my past. However, my body metabolized alcohol differently now.

When my mom offered to take the baby on the weekends, I went gangbusters. My weekends were anything but relaxing. During those weekends, I overindulged in everything. I socialized, slept very little, and was exhausted when I picked the baby up forty-eight hours later. I carried an emotional U-Haul of remorse, self-pity, doubt, and self-hate.

Depression crept in, and Mondays became unbearable with the baby. I stayed in bed and had a *down day*. I turned both the house and my cell phone to *do not disturb*, and I isolated myself. I told myself everything was okay. Afterall, no one was hurt, and we were home safe. I could not escape the tornado of depression, self-hate, and doubt. "As the feelings of hopelessness and depression progressed, so did my drinking." (The Big Book.)

Monday's mantra was common like a rewind from the week before. I promised myself, I won't ever do that again. Tuesdays brought relief when the sun rose and my headache faded. I was up and around the house. Wednesdays, I got up, got dressed, made dinner, and smiled. Thursdays felt great. I went to the gym and took a shower. On Fridays, the cycle started all over again. I'd put on my face and tennis shoes and pushed the stroller around the neighborhood. In the evenings, I mixed a martini and put it in my tumbler. All I wanted was to be married with a baby and stay home to raise her. So, why was I riding this emotional roller coaster? I had the picture-perfect life—a great husband, a home, cars, and social events to fill our weekends.

I wanted to control my drinking so badly, and I tried everything. Plagued by waves of self-pity and resentment, I wasn't doing too well at the time. Competing urges flooded me—*Drink! Just have one. No, don't drink! Drink this, not that, only drink with certain people*—it was so unsettling.

Making new rules for myself, I thought I could fix things by making small changes. *Switch from wine to vodka. Only drink on the weekends. Don't drink before 3:00 p.m. Blah Blah Blah.* Thank God my daughter won't remember any of this. For two years, I created so much chaos from drinking.

I felt alone with this baby. It felt more fun to raise her if I took the edge off with a glass of wine. I thought I would pull my ears off if I had to listen to one more *Yo Gabba Gabba!* song. A glass turned into a bottle of wine, which helped to smooth the high pitch sounds of the Disney channel and made me more playful.

"The idea that somehow, someday he will control and enjoy his drinking is the great obsession of every abnormal drinker. The persistence of this illusion is astonishing. Many pursue it into the gates of insanity or death." (The Big Book)

My husband drew a line in the sand. The last time I drank and drove with Liv in the car, he said, "It is my job to protect my kids, even if it mean us leaving you." I was not surprised to hear this. That is what a rational person would say. He had been my drinking partner for many years, but we were safe and not reckless. He did not have the alcoholic craving gene like I did. Jimmy used to be our driver before Uber was around. We had a lot of good times and carefree fun—but after pregnancy, everything shifted for me.

After this line-in-the-sand, I started to make even more excuses. Amid my insanity, I bought a two-seater sports car, so

I wouldn't have to drive anyone. Then, when Uber became an option, I frequently took advantage of it—way more than most people. When I drank with new acquaintances after my daughter's dance practice, I called an Uber to take the two of us home. She thought it was so cool when the black car arrived. I was using Uber to take us to her activities because I was drinking by 3:00 p.m. I made excuses like my car was in the shop. *Insanity.*

I had just finished a three-martini lunch at the Scottsdale Quarter, and my life was spinning in the wrong direction. Playing with fire every day, I got burned repeatedly, but this time, my actions left a lasting scar. The scar of affliction is now a badge of honor.

CHAPTER 4
QUIT THE INSANITY

HITTING BOTTOM

Rock bottom became the solid foundation
on which I rebuilt my life.

—J.K. Rowling

Hitting bottom is a term for when someone is ready to change their lives entirely. People often hit bottom when their privileges are taken away. It could mean losing their job or even losing their kids. Hitting bottom could come by killing someone in a car accident, taking a beating, giving a beating, repossession, foreclosure, losing a friend, divorce, and the list goes on. Everyone's bottom is different. When you reach the bottom (also known as your jumping off point), you have no doubt you've arrived. If you haven't hit bottom, then good for you because you figured out life quicker than most. I hope you never experience the dark side.

I AM SICK AND TIRED OF BEING SICK AND TIRED.

Staying insane was my safe place. I kept doing the same thing over and over hoping for a different result. Alcoholism is a thinking problem, not a drinking problem. I was safe in the prison between my ears. My insanity resulted in an unstable marriage, child endangerment, and instability, which included lying and being unreliable. I had reached my *jumping off point*. I am sick and tired of being sick and tired.

My last drunk driving was on Saint Patrick's Day, 2015. My husband was out of town traveling for business, which was normal for him. I went to meet a girlfriend at a steak house, not a place to drink green beer and be rowdy. It was a calm, sophisticated place. I told myself over and over again, *I dare not have a drink*, because I was driving, and my daughter was with me. I got to the Biltmore area restaurant after saying no the first two times to the server's request. But the third time, I said, "Yes. I'll have one." I was powerless over alcohol.

And then I had another. I could not say no to the second cold, dirty martini. We laughed and talked about my friend's latest swipe left.

The night came to an end, and I drove home. I had driven drunk once again with my kid in the car. My daughter was five years old at the time and didn't know any different than Mommy drinking with her friends. I put her to bed, and when I got to my room, I fell to my knees and asked for help. Pleading with God, I begged Him to show me a way to get out of this insanity. I had said many times before, *I am not doing that again*. But this time, something was different—I knew I needed help. I had a spiritual problem, and I needed a spiritual solution.

HUMBLE YOURSELVES BEFORE THE LORD, AND HE WILL LIFT YOU UP" (JAMES 4:10).

Humble yourselves before the Lord, and he will lift you up. (James 4:10).

Arizona is a no-tolerance state. I know a few people who have lost their kids or the privilege to drive them for a period of time because of a DUI, and I didn't want to be one of those parents. Drinking and driving on that holiday evening was my bottom.

After my pregnancy in 2010 and taking off time to breastfeed, alcohol was never the same for me. I continued to have blackouts after only a few drinks. Not only was I not emotionally present for my child, I also should have been locked up. It is only by the grace of God that I am alive today.

I knew of one neighbor on my street who didn't drink. One time, I'd asked her why she didn't drink as I pushed the stroller, looking for a happy hour drinking partner. She offered me only an iced tea. Louise was a former art gallery owner in Arizona and New Mexico who was now retired. She explained how she drank heavily for many years and now, not at all.

The following day was a typical, beautiful March day in Arizona, and I felt horrible about myself. Thoughts of self-hate filled my mind. I was thinking Liv might be better off without me, and I was lying to my husband again about my night out. While I stewed over the self-harming thoughts, I stood in the front yard pushing my daughter on the tree swing.

My neighbor Louise walked over. She was an older, stoic lady, and she was healthy with a tall, slender build. She always looked put together in her matching outfits—same material for the tops and bottoms. Most of the time, she looked as if she had walked off the cover of a Chico's catalog. She stopped by that day for a routine neighborly chat.

"How is Liv? Where is Michael traveling?" she quizzed.

God works in mysterious ways, and he must have put her in front of me that day. I cut the small talk and asked her, "How did you stop drinking?"

She didn't miss a beat and said, "It was not easy. Can you join me on Sunday at 5:00 p.m.? I'll tell you all about it. Show up at 4:30 p.m."

I showed up at Louise's beautifully decorated house. I glanced at the books on her coffee table. They were about art and French design. She was so interesting to me, so I was curious about her life.

She said, "Let's go."

I got in her full-size Cadillac and thought we were going for dinner—it was 4:30 p.m. on a Sunday evening, dinner time.

She drove toward Camelback Mountain. Some of my favorite fine restaurants were on the mountain with a sunset view. I thought it was going to be a good night.

We didn't go to a restaurant, though. She turned into a church in Paradise Valley and parked. We walked past the spacious main sanctuary all the way to the end of the campus where there was a large meeting room. The room was nice, with many chairs, and the air conditioner was cold. The faces were strangely familiar, though I didn't know anyone.

She said, "Welcome to your first Big Book meeting."

"Um … what?" That was *not* what I had expected. The court ordered meetings I attended twenty years ago were sad and depressing.

I had no idea what we were doing there, but on March 22, 2015, I willingly went to my first open A.A. meeting. Nervous about walking through those doors, I wondered, *What if someone sees me?* It seemed like everyone knew Louise. They came over and gave her hugs as she introduced me. Over and over I heard, "We are glad you're here." There was joy, chatting, and laughing in the room. People were hugging each other. I was really out of my comfort zone.

How are they so happy and not drinking? I was baffled as the self-proclaimed alcoholics had so much courage.

I have been drinking since the age of fourteen, so I didn't know how to socialize any other way.

As I walked in, a blast of cold air from the air conditioner hit my face. I was handed a ticket—was there going to be a raffle? I didn't see any prizes. Two men sat on tall chairs at the front of the room, with over one hundred chairs facing them. Everyone started filing in and finding seats. This was called a "speaker meeting," I learned.

The meeting started, and everyone introduced themselves with first name and sometimes, an adjective to follow. For example, Louise said, "Louise, grateful alcoholic." Others only gave their first names. There were also duel adjectives, like "Steve, alcohol and pills," or "Carrie, pills and sex." I was captivated by the speaker. His voice was hypnotizing. He was a former professional football player who shared his experience, strength, and hope. I couldn't believe the similarities in the thinking. A sober athlete. He referred to himself as infamous. In the meeting, he shared his story of how his life was unmanageable leading up to the biggest *draft bust* in the professional football history. *Well, if he can get sober and live to share about it*, I told myself, *I will give it my all*. "It was crystal clear. I wouldn't and couldn't drink anymore," (Mandarich, page 87). Plus, these people were kind of nice.

After he shared his story, they started calling numbers. If your number was called, you had the chance to speak and comment on what the speaker shared. So, that's what the tickets were for. The numbers were called one by one. Each person had two minutes to speak, so everyone had a chance to talk. They shared their experiences, relating to his story. These were my people—the brutal honesty that came from their mouths would have made most *normies* gasp. (Normie is a person who does not have a problem with alcohol and can enjoy it.) That room full of people had the same thoughts I did—sick and dark, self-defeating, regrets. I was drawn to their raw honesty. When the meeting ended, everyone joined hands and closed with the Lord's prayer. The prayer ended with a chant of "Keep coming back! It works if you work it."

I was silent until Louise broke the ice in the car. We had a great talk on the way home. I asked her, "What's the next step for me if I want to stop drinking?"

She said, "You? I didn't know you had a problem drinking. I thought you were here for someone else." She stopped herself, then she quickly replied, "Get a sponsor."

"What's a sponsor?" I asked.

"A sponsor," Louise said, "is who will walk you through the twelve-step program and be your most confident advisor."

"Will you be my sponsor?" I asked her.

She looked at me again, "Yes, I will help you. You will meet me weekly, and I will explain everything. Look on that smart phone of yours and find a meeting tomorrow. Then, call me." We arrived home, and I walked to my house across the street to join my family. I was unable to talk because I had to process everything I'd heard that day. It is also agreed upon that what goes on in the room stays in the room.

The next day, I went to my second meeting by myself to a not-so-fancy place. I walked through a cloud of cigarette smoke to find the front door. Someone greeted and welcomed me inside a fluorescent-lit room with a low popcorn ceiling. The linoleum squares on the floor were peeling. There were a couple of box fans blowing, but the room was hot and smelled like stale coffee and smoke. A podium stood tall in the front of the room, and on it was a symbol of a circle with a triangle inside of it. A table with three large metal coffee pots and piles of Styrofoam cups graced the left side of the room. A van pulled up, and a group of men with baggy jeans and tattoos got out and walked in the door. A waft of heat and body odor passed me by. I was shaking. *I don't belong here,* I thought to myself. But if that were true, then why did these stranger's faces seem so familiar to me?

I scanned the room for an empty folding chair and found a seat with the other women. One of them pushed The Big Book over to me to and said, "Follow along." The book was open to page fifty-eight, "Chapter 5: How it Works."

The meeting began. It had a similar format to the last meeting I attended with Louise. A person opened the meeting with the same jargon, and then another person talked for twenty minutes. Then, we had question and discussion time. The topic was Step 1.

Wait, I was on Step 1! *This is another sign I'm supposed to be here,* I thought, laughing to myself.

STEP 1: WE ADMITTED WE WERE POWERLESS OVER ALCOHOL—THAT OUR LIVES HAD BECOME UNMANAGEABLE.

Step 1: We admitted we were powerless over alcohol—that our lives had become unmanageable.

I admitted to myself that driving drunk and lying was my unmanageability, and when I drank, all bets were off. No matter what I planned, anything could happen, and I had no regard for rules or responsibility.

I stayed and listened to the meeting and what everyone shared for Step 1. Then, they gave me a list of meetings. There were hundreds of meetings daily, almost one every hour on the hour. I was in awe that the sober community was so big, and there were that many meetings.

I called Louise. "I went to a meeting," I told her. "It was scary."

"Great," she said. She must not have heard me. I explained again how scary the place was. Louise said calmly, "Look for the similarities, not the differences. Did you hear something that applied to you?" Then, it clicked. The meeting was scary not because I was in danger, but because I was back with the misfits of my childhood—back with the people I had tried so hard to leave behind.

"Yes," I said, "they were on Step 1." She said, "Go back tomorrow, Crystal. You need to stop everything and go to ninety meetings in ninety days. Your life depends on it."

"Ninety meetings in ninety days?" I asked in disbelief. "How am I supposed to do that?"

"Think of how much time you will have when you're not drinking," Louise said with a smile in her voice.

I sighed. "Okay, but how do I read this meeting list? What do all these abbreviations mean?"

Louise explained: "O is for *open meetings*, W is for *women's meetings*, M is for *men's meetings*, and S is for *speaker meetings*. C is for *closed meetings*, which are only for members and prospective members. SS is for *step studies*—where you study one of the 12 steps—and CC means there will be *childcare*. Now, get on that smartphone of yours and fill up your calendar."

I studied the meeting list and found a meeting to fit my schedule every day. There were so many meeting times right around the corner from my house. Lots of people were dealing with the same things. Once again, I felt like I was not alone. I was drawn toward the *closed meetings, women's meetings, and step studies*. However, I tried every type of meeting, and I heard parts of my story in each one I attended.

SUIT UP, SHOW UP, AND SHUT UP

Indeed, I went to ninety meetings in ninety days and visited Louise once a week at her house. She gave me homework and reset my expectation for myself. The first year I walked on eggshells. Isolated to the meetings and the people I had met there—I thought my life was over. I had no idea how I would stay married or see my drinking buddies again. How would I function in society if I couldn't drink? For so many years, alcohol had been my panacea: if I was happy, I would drink. If I was sad, I would drink. I definitely needed a drink to take the edge off before I attended a social event. It never entered my mind that I might have social anxiety because I was so full of alcohol-assisted confidence!

"People who conceal their sins will not prosper, but if they confess and turn from them, they will receive mercy" (Proverbs 28:13 NLT).

The *Pink Cloud* showed up, and I jumped on and held on with both hands.

I was a member of a new club, a secret society—the Book Club as we referred to it. I was a little skeptical, but I kept going back every day.

They said to me, "Can you just not drink today, and come back tomorrow?"

Everyone was so happy, nice, and welcoming. I attended mostly women's meetings, but my primary one was with child-care. I made that meeting my *home group*. (Your home group is where you get involved and start service work.)

My husband was glad I was not drinking and driving but was not happy I had traded in the booze for a group of people he didn't know. He didn't want me to label myself an alcoholic or stop drinking forever. "Couldn't you just take a break?" he'd ask. "Why do things have to be so extreme?" He didn't understand. His brain was not wired like mine. I knew I couldn't continue the same path any longer. I had to sacrifice everything to restore my sanity.

At the meetings, the optimism in the room was always unbelievable. I stared in amazement. *What are they so happy for? Aren't they alcoholics?*

For the first week or so of meetings, I didn't speak at all. I sat and listened … but mostly, I cried.

I sat in silence and continued to hear parts of my story from other women, realizing I was not the only one with the insane thoughts. The second week, I started to participate in the discussions. I still felt ashamed and defeated. When I spoke, I held back tears, and my voice cracked. It was about four weeks before I could smile.

Alcoholism is a thinking problem, not a drinking problem. Alcohol is but a symptom of a deeper issue. I thought getting sober would solve all my problems, and life would be easy, but I soon realized physical sobriety is only the first step—then comes emotional sobriety.

If you think your problems go away when you stop drinking, get ready. Now it is time to face them head-on. However, you don't need to do it alone. My sponsor walked me through each step and emotion.

With the exception of my husband, no one really knew I was going to meetings. I had talked to a few mom friends about my drinking and the consensus was, "I don't think you have a problem," and "Oh, don't be silly," and "You have a great life, just take the weekend off from drinking," go to Palm Springs and dry out" and other dismissive statements. I couldn't tell them I had tried all of that, and none of it worked. I was to the point where I hid my drinking at home.

I heard all of my stories in the rooms. I realized there was nothing I could tell Louise, my most trusted advisor, that would shock her. When I told Louise all of my deepest, darkest thoughts, she still showered me with love and grace.

STEP 5: ADMITTED TO GOD, TO OURSELVES, AND TO ANOTHER HUMAN BEING THE EXACT NATURE OF OUR WRONGS. (THE BIG BOOK)

Step 5: Admitted to God, to ourselves, and to another human being the exact nature of our wrongs. (The Big Book)

Taking emotional inventory is the hardest, most self-enlightening thing I've ever done. The intention is to examine each of your character defects, then confess them to God and another human being with honesty. It was very hard and time consuming, but when it was complete it was the most spiritual thing I have ever experienced. Physically, it felt like I took a huge weight off my back.

I completed ninety days of sobriety, attended ninety meetings, and worked the twelve steps with Louise, I began to feel lighter, like a real person again. I started to feel I would be a good mother, and I started to enjoy my secret community. The anonymity of it was thrilling. I loved to see people from my daughter's school, church, and the health club referring to it as *a spotting in the wild.* We gave each other a discreet nod and a smile and kept on walking.

What once kept me isolated and alone had now given me the keys to the kingdom. My darkness had become my shining light. Once I knew who I was and what my purpose was, I was free to serve others by sharing my experience, strength, and hope. Alcohol brought me to *The Big Book*, and the steps brought me to God.

Before I found the step-by-step recovery program, I believed it was best to leave the past in the past. While reading the *Big Book*, I found a simple program for complicated people.

Ask yourself, *Do you have an addiction? Is something holding you back from becoming your best self?* The remarkable thing about this recovery program is its applicability to any vice—pills, food, narcotics, smoking, overeating, gambling, sex addiction, the list goes on. Once you work and hone the steps, you, too, can become a Peaceful Warrior.

Take this time to pause and reflect. Is recovery right for you? We strive for progress, not perfection. It is a program designed not for those who *need it* but for those who *want it.*

I know why we're here.
We're all here because we're not all there.

—Steven Tyler

DID YOU KNOW?

Only you can decide whether you want to give recovery a try. We who are in recovery came because we finally gave up trying to control our drinking. We still hated to admit that we could never drink safely. Then we heard that we were sick. (We thought so for years!) We found out that many people suffered from the same feelings of guilt and loneliness and hopelessness that we did. We found out that we had these feelings because we had the disease of alcoholism.

We decided to try and face up to what alcohol had done to us. Here are some of the questions we tried to answer honestly. If we answered YES to four or more questions, we were in deep trouble with our drinking.

Answer YES or NO to the following twelve questions.

1. Have you ever decided to stop drinking for a week or so, but only lasted for a couple of days?

2. Do you wish people would mind their own business about your drinking—stop telling you what to do?

3. Have you ever switched from one kind of drink to another in the hope that this would keep you from getting drunk?

4. Have you had to have an eye-opener upon awakening during the past year?

5. Do you envy people who can drink without getting into trouble?

6. Have you had problems connected with drinking during the past year?

7. Has your drinking caused trouble at home?

8. Do you ever try to get "extra" drinks at a party because you do not get enough?

9. Do you tell yourself you can stop drinking any time you want to, even though you keep getting drunk when you don't mean to?

10. Have you missed days of work or school because of drinking?

11. Do you have "blackouts"?

12. Have you ever felt that your life would be better if you did not drink?

RESULTS

Did you answer YES four or more times? If so, you are probably in trouble with alcohol.

See Appendix II in the back of the book for more in-depth explanation.

CHAPTER 5
QUIT SITTING ON THE PEDESTAL

SOBER SISTERS ON A PINK CLOUD

We strive for progress, not perfection.

—*The Big Book*

I was riding what is referred to as the *pink cloud* because I was sober. Louise and two of my treasured sober sisters celebrated my one-year anniversary of sobriety with me over lunch at Arcadia Farms. They gave me a thread bracelet with a charm, a triangle—our secret society symbol—and a blingy one-year chip. My husband called and secretly paid the bill. I could not believe I had completed a year of sobriety, which changed everything. This made me feel that I was a good wife, mother, sister, and friend.

Because I had reconciled my past, I felt as though I was walking on air. I was part of a secret society and had it all figured out. *The 9th Step Promises* had come true on page 83 & 84 of The Big Book.

1. If we are painstaking about this phase of our development, we will be amazed before we are halfway through.

2. We are going to know a new freedom and a new happiness.

3. We will not regret the past nor wish to shut the door on it.

4. We will comprehend the word serenity and we will know peace.

5. No matter how far down the scale we have gone, we will see how our experience can benefit others.

6. That feeling of uselessness and self-pity will disappear.

7. We will lose interest in selfish things and gain interest in our fellows.

8. Self-seeking will slip away.

9. Our whole attitude and outlook upon life will change.

10. Fear of people and of economic insecurity will leave us.

11. We will intuitively know how to handle situations which used to baffle us.

12. We will suddenly realize that God is doing for us what we could not do for ourselves.

Are these extravagant promises? We think not. They are being fulfilled among us-sometimes quickly, sometimes slowly. They will always materialize if we work for them.

My life could not have been any better. I had mended my marriage, and we celebrated our tenth anniversary with a happy, healthy weekend away at Havasupai Falls. We hiked and enjoyed the beauty of the outdoors. I appreciated parenthood with my daughter, and I started to get my footing back and decided to go back to work. Also, I got involved at my daughter's school as the room mom. I was social again, and I was at peace being in any environment. These words from *The Big Book* were true for me: "We are not fighting it, neither are we avoiding temptation. We feel as though we had been placed in a position of neutrality—safe and protected. We have not even sworn off. Instead, the problem has been removed. It does not exist for us."

The Big Book restored my sanity. Life was very good. I was stable and happy as was everyone around me. I began to get busy with life and taught fitness classes at the local health club and spa. Slowly, the thought, *I have been cured,* crept in my mind. *I am no longer an alcoholic! Look how long I have been sober.* These were dangerous thoughts, as I soon discovered.

I got my eighteen-month chip. I was coasting, feeling confident with my head held high. April rolled around, and the weather felt perfect. I thought everything was going well. My two years was a few months away, so why not enjoy myself with an iced-cold drink? One sunny day, after weeks of contemplation, I had a drink at a spring-training game. I was with a group of girls on the executive level with the open bar, and I felt okay after the first drink. *That wasn't so bad,* I thought. *I'll have another.* Once I had the second drink, and then another, my old behavior reared its ugly head. My character was gone, and the person I didn't recognize came out. I got home safely that night, but I knew I hadn't made my sober self-proud of my conversation or conduct that day.

The next weekend, I had three drinks over two days. The following week, I started on Thursday. I was right back where I left off. I didn't see this as a relapse but a conscious choice to drink again. I had thought about it for weeks before it happened, I knew I wasn't drinking out of spite or anger. Three weeks of the insane drinking and thinking and I was on my knees again, pleading for help. I was ashamed to go back to the meetings, thinking, *I let everyone down.* When I returned sobbing, they said, "We don't shoot our wounded," and I was welcomed back with open arms. I felt my shame lift away, and I went right back into the steps.

Then, something strange happened. Like my stillbirth, no one talks about it until you are going through it. They welcomed me with open arms when I shared my shame. They inundated me with stories of relapses and how it is part of the journey to understand your disease completely.

"We are not cured of alcoholism. What we really have is a daily reprieve contingent on the maintenance of our spiritual condition. Every day we must carry the vision of God's will into all of our activities." *(The Big Book)*

Louise's health was failing being well over the age of eighty. She recommended I get a new sponsor. The way to find a sponsor is to go to meetings, listen, and find someone you relate to. I quickly got back into service work and out of my head.

I joined the committee to procure a conference in Phoenix in 2017. The conference was for female recovering alcoholics from across the world. Phoenix won the bid, and we entered the planning mode for the conference. It was a two-year monthly service commitment.

At one of the committee meetings, I heard a woman laugh from across the room. There were a hundred women in the room, but I noticed her joy right away. I approached her and asked her to be my sponsor. We were both serving on the conference committee. She said she would meet with me.

Her name was Sandy Simon. Very well put together, she looked like the actress, Sharon Stone. She was very statuesque. She had raised three boys and had been sober for over twenty years. Her husband had just passed away, and he had been an executive like my husband was. When Sandy stopped drinking, he had not, but she was still able to stay married. Many marriages fall apart when one spouse gets sober, and I was afraid mine would, too. I hoped she could teach me how to save my marriage.

As much as I wanted to stay married, I also want to create an identity of my own, separate from my husband. Sandy had done that, too. She had two jobs, one as an airline flight attendant and one in a retail store. Both of those jobs were part-time. With alcoholic and sober friends all over the country, her role as a flight attendant allowed her to visit them whenever she liked. She lived down the street from me, but she was often away from home, jetting off to visit one of her many friends scattered across the United States. I thought that was the coolest thing. She was a wife and mother like me, but now that she had raised her children, she was living her life and loving it. I wanted to know how I could do that, too.

Most of all, Sandy had joy! She had what I wanted, not only physical sobriety but *emotional sobriety*, too. Sandy coached me on how to *get it* and *keep it* while staying married and raising kids. She enjoyed life, had a contagious laugh and smile, and hugged everyone. I wanted to imitate her, and I was elated about acquiring this new-found emotional sobriety.

I recapped my previous week when I met with Sandy each week, quick to say how I *should have* this or *should have* that. Saying it out loud to someone else, I immediately heard how I should have handled a situation in a better way.

She stopped me abruptly. "Don't *should* on yourself. To know better is to do better. So, *do* better next time."

Marveling at Sandy's cut-to-the-chase attitude, I admired her.

Boundaries and knowing thy self are an ever-evolving process that comes with time management. It involves self-care and a clear head when you commit to doing something. As moms, we often want always to say yes and be supermoms. If you don't accept the commitment with the right intentions, it will backfire and end up draining you (and your time).

Sandy was the best sounding board. "What's on your mind this week?" she'd ask.

I'd list the opportunities I had to help at the school PTO. She reminded me of the service commitments I already had. "You don't have time for that," she said. "You have several plates spinning, and if you continue to add more plates, you will drop one."

She looked me in the eyes. "You don't want to drop one. Do you?" I mean, so many of us are constantly juggling.

I shook my head.

She said, "You cannot take on any more plates. Reply with, thank you for the invitation. I cannot at this time."

I must have looked unconvinced. She quickly followed up with, "What others think of you is not your business." And boom, problem solved.

Sandy and I met every week for roughly two years. She poured into me all of her wisdom and serenity, stressing the importance of having emotional support from your female friends because most men's love language is *the provider* not emotional support. I knew this about mine from reading *The 5 Love Languages.*

She was taken too soon by small-cell lung cancer. Sandy was special. She was one of those people who Kary Oberbrunner writes about in *Your Secret Name:* "Such people have a restorative quality about them. Rather than taking energy from others, they're so full of life that they give energy to others." "The end of all things is near. Therefore, be alert and of sober mind so that you may pray." (1 Peter 4:7)

PART 2

QUIT SHUTTING THE DOOR ON YOUR EMOTIONS

Now that I have shared my stories with you, I will share how I put everything I learned into action. If you choose sobriety, how do you maintain it? How do you learn to feel again after numbing yourself for so many years? How do you choose spiritual fitness every day? I will show you how in Part Two.

CHAPTER 6

QUIT USING OTHER PEOPLE'S VERSIONS OF GOD

THE SPIRITUAL SIDE OF SOBRIETY

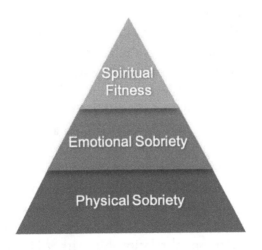

According to the *Many Paths to Spirituality*, "My sponsor encouraged me to choose my own conception of a higher power. It did not have to be a gender, or a name, or any human attributes—it just had to be 'a power greater than myself.' It was then I realized the fellowship, though comprised of human beings, represented a power greater than anything human. Even more surprisingly, by taking the Steps in my own clumsy way, supported by the unconditional love of my fellow alcoholics, I had discovered a quiet, inner voice—a God within."

This made sense to me. I was able to compare it to my softball background in this way:

When watching the All-American past time, baseball, the audience roots for the batter to get a hit and advance to first base. Did you know that there are seven ways to get on first base? That's right, seven different ways to accomplish the same thing. It's not so important how they get there but that they arrive at the first base.

Finding a higher power is very similar—there are many different ways to get there. Maybe you did not grow up in church, or maybe you grew up in a catholic church with a punishing God. Whatever your idea of God is, finding a high power is simply believing in something bigger than yourself.

There is often some confusion about the relationship between religion and spirituality. The Marine Corp's position towards spiritual fitness is a philosophy I can relate to. Their online handbook explains that religion and spirituality are completely interconnected, while for others they are distinct. Though opinions vary and for each individual, they may have unique meanings. For the sake of clarity, the concepts of religion and spirituality will be treated as separate but often related constructs. Religion is an organized set of beliefs and practices adhered to by a group of people. It is practiced externally with the intent to foster spirituality. Spirituality is an internal experience. It is characterized by one's personal experience of meaning, connection, and transcendence. It may include a personal relationship with a Higher Power or a purpose that gives meaning to life. Research shows that religion can be an effective way to foster the benefits of spirituality because it provides teachings, scripture, rituals, and practices that can enhance personal meaning, direction, connection, and fulfillment. However, just being part of a religion does not make a person "spiritual." It is also possible to be a spiritual person without being religious, or even believing in God as defined by religion. For many people who are not religious, spirituality is about living in harmony with nature and society. Others use a powerful principle as their guiding source of inspiration, such as love, patriotism, truth, or the human spirit. Many seek to understand and develop their own "higher self." Whether you choose to use religion or choose to follow a different path, the key to developing spirituality is to make regular sincere efforts to find deeper connection and meaning in your life.

(To read the full article, go to, https://www.hqmc.marines.mil/Agencies/Marine-Corps-Spiritual-Fitness/Spiritual-Fitness-Tie-ins-Copy/)

WHAT IS EMOTIONAL SOBRIETY?

I hear this question when I use the hashtag in my social media posts #emotionalsobriety. Someone who is emotionally sober is the opposite of a dry drunk. In case you haven't heard the term, *dry drunk*, it is someone who stopped drinking but remained miserable. Emotional sobriety is not only sobriety on a physical level, but also in your thoughts and actions. For

> EMOTIONAL INTELLIGENCE IS THE ABILITY TO MAINTAIN YOUR CHARACTER DESPITE THE CIRCUMSTANCES.

addicts, emotional intelligence does not come naturally. *Emotional intelligence is the ability to maintain your character despite the circumstances.* It is to be sober in your thoughts to pause and respond but not react haphazardly. I didn't learn that in school or from my parents. I learned it from my spiritual advisor. Emotional sobriety is necessary to live in joy. The daily tools I use to remain in emotional sobriety are The Serenity Prayer and self-care. When I practice the *Power Hour* and give my will over to God, the rest of the day falls into place. You may have heard the old cliché, "One day at a time," but it really works. As another saying goes, "Yesterday is history, tomorrow is a mystery, and today is a gift. That's why it is called the present." Living emotionally sober is as simple as giving your will over to God and doing the next right thing.

GARBAGE IN, GARBAGE OUT

"You look great. What are you training for?" I often hear this question at my health club and in my circle of mom friends. When I respond with, "I am training for *life*," I see the curiosity on their faces. What does it mean to train for life? It means to get up every day and enjoy life, including a routine. I hear moms say, "I can't wait to get through the day (or the week)," or, "I am so glad school started (or finished)." It seems like no matter what season they are in, they are unsettled, waiting for the next season to start. Last summer, at our church's summer camp for kids, Pastor Ryan talked about GIGO. It could not have been any more straightforward for me. This is why I like children's bible study because I am an infant when it comes to understanding the bible. GIGO stands for "garbage in, garbage out," and it was originally a computer term. But Pastor Ryan applied it to our brains as he taught the kids about what we fill our minds with. Alcoholism is a thinking problem, not a drinking problem. So, I must constantly check my thoughts. I have to be careful of what I listen to—I don't want to listen to complaints or victim attitudes. I am a victor *over* this disease, not a victim *of* it. If a worst-case scenario runs through my head for more than ten minutes, I know to pick up the phone and call someone. They help me sort out my thoughts to see what my part in the situation was. This mind exercise has saved me many days and nights of worry. "Worrying is like meditating on shit." (Movie quote from *Thank You for Sharing, 2012*). I no longer have to worry about what is out of my control. As Sandy would say, "Sounds like you are in the solution, not the problem."

POWER HOUR

I adopted the FIT Power Hour from Kim Dolan Leto, author of *F.I.T.: Faith Inspired Transformation*. She explains how her time with God in the morning gives her more time in the day. I could not agree more. Applying these simple steps keeps me emotionally sober and very humble. It breaks down like this.

Fit Soul—Time in the Word
Fit Mind—Time in reflection, prayer, and gratitude
Fit Body—Time exercising

Spend twenty minutes on each part, and make it a habit to practice self-care. If you don't take care of yourself—soul, mind, and body—you are no good to your family. Your family and friends will thank you for it.

Now, if I get the RID's restless, irritable, and discontent (which still does happen), I can recover from it more quickly. The tool I use is HALT: I stop to see if I am *hungry, angry, lonely,* or *tired*. 99% of the time, the root of my bad mood is one of these. When I was a young wife, one of my common complaints was feeling lonely all the time. I thought having a baby would solve that. It did not. Now that I have had a spiritual awakening, I realize I am never alone because God is walking with me. I was lonely because I didn't have a relationship with God.

Start your day off with a prayer. Here are my three favorite prayers from the *Big Book*.

Morning Prayer

God, direct my thinking today so that it be empty of self-pity, dishonesty, self-will, self-seeking, and fear. God, inspire my thinking, decisions, and intuitions. Help me to relax, and take it easy. Free me from doubt and indecision. Guide me through this day, and show me my next step. God, show me what I need to do to take care of any problems. I ask all of these things that I maybe of maximum service to you and my fellow man.

Night Prayer

God, forgive me where I have been resentful, selfish, dishonest, or afraid today. Help me to not keep anything to myself but to discuss it all openly with another person—show me where I owe an apology and help me make it. Help me to be kind and loving to all people. Use me in the mainstream of life, God. Free me of worry, remorse, or morbid (sick) reflections that I may be of usefulness to others. AMEN.

Serenity Prayer

God grant me the serenity to accept the things I cannot change, the courage to change the things I can, and the wisdom to know the difference.

I sit down on Sunday nights and prepare for our weekly family meetings. On the whiteboard calendar in our living room, I write each family member's activities for the week, what night we will have family dinners, what will I make for dinner at home, and my FIT hour. Sometimes, the small planning session takes ten minutes, sometimes thirty. I go over every hour of my day and make sure I will be exactly where I should be. Success can come from what you *don't* do. An invitation to go for coffee or lunch is flattering, but if this makes your day rushed, or if the person drains you instead of filling you up, it is okay to say, no thank you.

SPIRITUAL FITNESS

It is not uncommon for best friends, partners, or spouses to get upset with you when you don't drink. You used to be their drinking buddy for many years. It's common to hear things like, "We did not invite you to the concert because you have that thing." That *thing* they're referring to is your commitment to staying sober which makes them uncomfortable. Hearing these statements baffled me when I started to develop spiritual fitness, but now I can handle them with grace.

> SPIRITUAL FITNESS IS WHEN YOU CAN GO ANYWHERE, IN ANY SITUATION, AND NOT FALL INTO YOUR OLD PATTERNS.

Emotional sobriety is being mindful of and sober in your thoughts. *Spiritual Fitness is when you can go anywhere, in any situation, and not fall into your old patterns.* It is your resistance to outside influences and remaining strong in your faith and values. When you aren't emotionally sober, you can't become spiritually fit. Spiritual fitness gives you the strength to maintain your emotional sobriety. It's your resistance to outside influences. Whether you're at a bar or a church potluck, if you're spiritually fit, you can be yourself and have a good time.

Here are some Spiritually Fit responses to situations you might find yourself in:

Q: *Do you want a drink?* A: *No, thanks, I see someone I want to say hi to.*

Q: *What can I get you to drink?* A: *You're busy hosting. I'll get my own, thanks.*

Q: *Here, have the cocktail of the night.* A: *Oh, where's the restroom? I'll get it when I come back.*

Q: *Are you ever going to be able to drink again?* A: *Not sure, but today I will pass.*

Q: *When are we going to have a drink together?* A: *Call me tomorrow.* (They always forget, and *tomorrow* never comes.)

I find that morning stretch and breath is also a great way for me to stay spiritually fit:

Show up on your mat and be still. Find your breath. Ground yourself. Stretch further, then relax into the posture. Breathing while stretching is restraining the natural turbulence of thought. When you spend time on your mat, several things happen. The teacher instructs you to move your body, so you don't have to think about it. You are left alone with your thoughts, and many thoughts will surface while you are quiet for ninety minutes. The teacher's voice will fade into the background while the body moves to the words. What is heavy on the mind, good or bad, will come out of the heart during practice, and your perspective will change. The fact that you showed up on your mat and stayed for the entire time will give you the mental strength to process your feelings. This small act of physical and mental discipline will bring out your inner warrior who is well prepared for whatever life brings you. The warrior will do the next right thing with love and compassion. You will not only get through life, but you will *enjoy* life.

I love Glennon Doyle Melton's simple definition of a warrior:

What I Know: 1. What you don't know, you're not supposed to know yet. 2. More will be revealed. 3. Crisis means to sift. Let it all fall away and you'll be left with what matters. 4.What matters most cannot be taken away. 5. Just do the next right thing one thing at a time. That'll take you all the way home.

—Glennon Doyle Melton, *Love Warrior*

What does a spiritually fit life look like? Commemorating life's milestones with something other than alcohol can be tricky, but it's possible. Scheduling monthly date nights with my husband has been one of our values as a couple. I went from addicted, isolated weekends, to much richer ones full of socializing, celebrating our time together with or without friends, or food-centered events. We enjoy couples' massages, pedicures, a comedy show, buying a special candle, taking a long bath, or listening to books on tape and then discussing them. Celebrating the chaos of life together is what we relish in. Nothing is too big or small to handle. When we are spiritually fit, we welcome the waves of life like a surfer on the North Shore. Be Holy. "Therefore, with minds that are alert and fully sober, set your hope on the grace to be brought to you when Jesus Christ is revealed at his coming" (1 Peter 1:13).

CHAPTER 7
QUIT DEPENDING ON OTHERS FOR YOUR JOY

HAPPINESS IS A CHOICE

John 16:22 says, *"No one will take away your joy."* You control your joy. Nothing can remove your joy unless you give it away. There is a spiritual crisis in the land of the free and home of the brave. People from many other countries are dying to get into the United States of America. So, why do we take our physical freedom and spiritual fitness for granted? What was the American dream for freedom is now a dream of having more: if I only had a bigger house, newer cars, longer vacations. You have everything you need right inside of you. The important things cannot be taken away. Ignite your flame.

Life is not good or bad; it just is. My husband is hands-down the best at applying this principle to his life. He embodies the young spirit of an entrepreneur, and that lifestyle comes with highs and lows. It's how you respond to it that really matters. It took me a long time to figure this out. Now that I have all the right emotional and spiritual tools in my toolbox, I can travel anywhere with anyone, and enjoy what life offers in any situation. My favorite spiritual fitness tool is the ability to routinely pause and *respond* instead of *reacting*. Another great tool is the ten-minute rule: Will this matter in ten minutes, ten days, or ten years from now? And I respond accordingly.

Life will continue to get, for the lack of a better term, *lifey*. The health of your parents will decline, children will continue to evolve with successes and failures, and friends will let you down. In the past, I wasn't able to see the joy in life during these times, and I numbed it by drinking. Life sent me into a *fuck it* spiral. Alcohol was such a socially acceptable coping balm. I would say to myself, "If only (fill in the blank), then I could be happy." Now, with my Spiritual toolbox, I can *Pause*, *Pray*, and *Plan* my reaction, take myself through the processing steps, and have a completely different outlook on the situation. My mantra is: *This, too, shall pass*. Life's moments—the good and the bad—are temporary. It is a choice to *be in the solution, not the problem*.

My daughter started dancing at four years old. The dance class was more for the moms to socialize and pass the time, rather than for rigorous dance training. It was a fun space, air-conditioning for the moms, and make-up and costumes for the girls. In my younger days, softball brought me a lot of pain, physically and emotionally. I was conscious about guiding my daughter to an indoor sport with more glamorous gear than a glove and a ball. Softball was brutal with sweat, bruises, and dirt. I was also mindful of spending weekends on the soccer field or softball field. It became like a camping experience, hauling in shade and water, and every piece of equipment to make the kids comfortable in the outdoors. When we rode our bikes past the neighborhood softball park, and I cringed, I no longer saw the joy in it.

So, my daughter danced at a studio with the best studio owner, Miss Annie. She was camera-ready every day. When we walked in the studio, Annie gave Liv a big hug and made her feel like a million bucks with her welcoming smile. There were over one hundred girls in the dance studio throughout the course of an evening, but Miss Annie made each one feel special. To pass the time, the moms would either go shopping, sip margaritas at the local Mexican food joint, or hang in the studio and gossip. I met some of my closest friends at Liv's dance class. However, no matter what was happening in the studio—with politics, teachers, parents, or girls—Miss Annie always greeted us with a smile. She exuded happiness in her teaching—the same amount of happiness every day. Her love for the little ones showed that she had such passion for what she did. One day, she sent out an email regarding controversial teacher turnover and how it was handled. When I walked in the studio that day, there was low rumbling of speculation and gossip. I turned to Annie and said, "How are you always happy?" She quickly responded, "Happiness is a choice," and flashed her pearly whites into a grin with a wink. I loved her keep your head up so your crown doesn't fall off attitude.

> KEEP YOUR HEAD UP SO YOUR CROWN DOESN'T FALL OFF.

Wow, so simple but so profound. I mean who has time to get frown lines? Miss Annie is my hero—with such a big heart. She was the perfect weight and long blonde hair. She lived out her dream of dancing and teaching little girls to find their confidence, character, and poise. No matter how *lifey* life got, she *showed up filled up.*

Spiritual fitness is a journey, not a destination. Slow down and revel in the Holy Spirit.

VICTIMS VS. VICTORS

In fitness studios all over the valley, while teaching and practicing, I have witnessed miracles firsthand. You are never too late, too sick, or too old to start practicing self-care. Life comes with crossroads. When you receive *bad* news of a failing health condition such as little Joey's ADHD or your parents' failing health, you can take one of two roads. There is Victim Avenue—the mindset that life is happening to you and is out of your control—or Victor Boulevard—the mindset that life is simply happening, and you can remain in joy and learn from the lesson. Which road will you take, Victim Avenue or Victor Boulevard?

One day, while I was teaching hot yoga, a man in his mid-forties walked in. He was a cross-country truck driver and had decided to give up his career because it was killing him. At least fifty pounds overweight, he had a hard belly that hung over his belt. His legs were reddish-purple from the knee down due to circulation issues, and he was on a buffet of medications. He had hit his rock bottom. His approach was simple—he was going to change everything. The goal of the first day in class is to stay in the room. I sat up a chair for him in the back of the room, and his mat was in front of the chair. He stayed in the chair and did his stretching from a seated position. He returned every day for thirty days. A week into his practice, he was able to remove the chair and get up and down from the mat. Barely able to stand on one foot, he held onto the wall to support himself. The second week, he continued to lean on the wall for support. The third week, he moved to the second row and balanced on both feet with his arms over his head. I watched as he showed up every day and did his best. The purple-red color on his legs started to diminish, and his waistline was going down. His faith was unwavering, and he restored his health and his quality of life.

CHAPTER 8
QUIT EATING EMPTY CALORIES

EAT TO LIVE, DON'T LIVE TO EAT

The food you eat can be either the safest and most powerful
form of medicine or the slowest form of poison.

—Ann Wigmore

As a kid, I woke up on Saturday mornings to the smell of
sausage and biscuits. I'd grab an extra-large, golden-canned
biscuit, pull apart the flaky crisped dough, place it on a
plate, and lift the ladle. My mouth would water. I'd scoop the
gravy and pour it over the biscuit as I watched the white gravy
with lumps of sausage ooze onto the biscuits. Cutting another
biscuit in half, I'd lather on the butter and jelly. I thought I was
the luckiest kid in the world with such delicious, homemade food
for breakfast. Little did I know, the home cooking was creating
the layer of fat that would cover my body.

I was never overweight by the standard guidelines, but *thick*,
as I heard in high school. With more muscle than most girls,
I still had a layer of fat covering my legs and arms. I was very
self-conscious about my weight and body shape. I had to con-
tinually wear a belt because of my small waist and big hips, so I
tried every diet: *The Grapefruit Diet, Body for Life*, deprivation,
removing whole food groups, counting calories and carbohydrates,

macros, and the list goes on. The only way I knew how to maintain my weight was with food obsession. I did this when training for a fitness-stage show, a race, an athletic competition, or simply to feel great in a gorgeous dress on a Friday night out. I was either on or off a food plan—there was no middle ground. And I'd go into a tailspin of indecision when I visited a restaurant. I'd study the menu with precision, but even when I thought I'd ordered perfectly, I'd wake up the next day with puffy eyes because of the high salt content in the restaurant food. Those puffy eyes reminded me of how sensitive my body was but also how in touch I was with my body. The security of physical then emotional sobriety has allowed me to live at a healthy weight and change my perspective on food. I now celebrate it as one of life's gifts.

While writing this book, several people close to me were diagnosed with cancer. The movie *Fork over Knife,* changed my perspective on meat in relationship to cancer. The movie and Dr. Esselstyn, M.D., showed studies that everyone is predisposed with cancer cells, but he demonstrated how eating less than 2% of calories from meat can turn *off* cancer cells. We are all born with the cancer genes, and whether we turn them on or off are based on our choices, lifestyle, and environment. Obesity recently surpassed smoking as the number one leading cause of preventable cancer. A new study presented at the Society of General Internal Medicine's 2017 Annual Meeting found that obesity has caused up to 47% more life-years lost than tobacco. The authors also found that tobacco-related life years lost were similar to the rate of hypertension. https://www.pharmacytimes. com/news/obesity-responsible-for-more-deaths-than-smoking

It is a known fact that not smoking reduces the chance of lung cancer. Now, we know that poor food choice increases the chance of preventable cancer. Maintaining an ideal body weight reduces the chance of dying from lifestyle choice disease. What I know is that dis + ease = disease. Inflammation causes disease, and wrong foods cause inflammation.

Understanding how to *live to eat* and not *eat to live* is a conscious shift. Continued overeating can lead to a slow and painful death. What a miserable life it would be if we were unable to put on shorts and chase our kid at the splash pad. It would be sad not to join your husband at an event because you don't feel confident enough. If you are missing out on life because of your body image, it is up to you to change it. In this case, your success can come from what you don't eat.

If you fail to plan, you plan to fail - I have been here before with alcohol. Instead of *when I will drink next?* it is: *What won't I eat next?* This is a miserable way to live with that loud food noise. Enjoying food and cutting out the chaos can be manageable and enjoyable.

Sometimes, people can have dual addictions when one substance is absent, but there are still problems. It is common as a beginner to think, *I don't have a problem with alcohol. I will just stop the pills*—or pot—or whatever the other substance is. This is also called a cross-addiction.

I heard early on in my recovery to be careful because when you stop drinking, your body may continue to crave sugar, and you could add on some weight. The joke was, "You can't get arrested for eating a Snickers bar—so give some grace and some chocolate." I was very conscious not to do this and just drink water.

Applying recovery tricks to food does not completely work because you cannot abstain from food. My spiritual fitness has allowed me to develop a method of eating that is very satisfying.

First, I figure out how many meals I need for the week. We sit down for a quick Sunday night family meeting to review activities, including when we can have a family dinner, and also when it will be a homemade meal. Then, I decide what we will eat for the week. That determines my grocery list. My neighborhood grocery store has a great mobile app that allows me to order food by scanning containers I already have. I scan empty food containers before throwing them away, ensuring I always have the staples of my kitchen. My favorite and must-have staples in the kitchen are Pink Himalayan salt and cracked black pepper. Eating mostly plant-based meals has cut back on my refined oils, which I used to love to buy. The riper the food, the less oil it needs. Oil isn't bad on its own, but refined oils are often chemically altered, so I use sparingly.

Here is a simple plan to cut chaos out of the kitchen:

1. Plan your meals: how many meals will you and your family have at home this week? Include breakfast, lunch, and dinner.

2. Plan the menu: review your recipes and choose which ones to make.

3. Order groceries online and schedule pick up or delivery time.

4. Sharpen your knives and gather glass jars and containers.

5. Prep meals for the week.

6. Prep snacks for the week.

7. Grab and Go

8. Enjoy your food!

The Blessing

Asking God to bless the food before the meal has been an accepted ritual handed down from generation to generation. It has been thought by some to promote better nutrition and healing by raising the vibration of the food. Better that we ask God to bless our proper selection of more complete foods as we go shopping for that which will advance our physical and our spiritual needs.

—Stanley Burroughs

First, I order my groceries online. I do a quick kitchen inventory of what I have, and the app allows me to look at my meals and order exactly what I need to make them. Ordering groceries on the app has cut down on our grocery bill by reducing impulse buying and applying electronic coupons based on what I put in my cart. Going to the grocery store unprepared is a miserable experience with so many choices and lots of distractions. The ability to pick up my groceries at curbside is exactly what I need. Ironically, ordering online—although a sedentary activity—restores my health and gives me more time and money. The time I used to spend pushing the cart down the aisles is time I now spend chopping up fresh fruit, veggies, seeds, and nuts.

When I arrive home from the grocery store, I lay out all my veggies and get ready to prep. I put on some music, sharpen the knives, and grab the cutting boards. Food prepping is as simple as washing, chopping, and portioning. I roast vegetables and portion them into glass jars for my lunches. I like to use glass jars because they are the perfect size for my stomach. Also, heating up in glass is better for you than reheating plastic Tupperware, which has been known to leak carcinogens and free radicals into the food. A jar full of superfood with beneficial calories satisfies me and gives me the energy I need. You should not spend more than two hours prepping food.

While enjoying a great summer and sharing a beach house with our extended family, we decided to take turns making dinner. The dinners were all delicious but watching how people felt after the dinner was an eye-opener. When my family ate pasta with red sauce, I witnessed their heartburn and indigestion. They celebrated nightly with ice cream, only to be unsettled the next morning about overindulging or feeling too full.

For as long as I can remember, my mother talked about people's weight, constantly pointing out how their clothes didn't fit them properly, how their bellies hung over their belts, or how their gait was at a slower pace.

She would say, "As long as you stay thin, you avoid a ton of health problems, and you can shop anywhere." It was a big deal in my family when my stepdad's waistline grew over thirty-eight inches because he no longer found clothes that fit him at the *regular* department stores. This was before retailers carried sizes like XXXL on their racks. Being super-sized nowadays is no longer an inconvenience. You can shop at Walmart or Old Navy with the rest of the family and still buy the latest trend—only in a larger size. My mother verbalized she didn't accept his size, but he still overindulged.

But my mother was a food pusher, which contributed to my stepfather's lifestyle-harbored disease and led to his death at the early age of sixty-four. Then, she turned into the food police on a dime. "Don't eat the banana bread! Don't eat that; eat this instead." It was culinary whiplash.

My stepdad death certificate had a long list of organs that had failed. His health decline started around the age of forty with a diabetes diagnosis while on one pill. That one pill had a side effect of high blood pressure which required yet another pill. Then, the coumadin came along with the daily shots. The big pharmaceutical companies failed him. He believed that their drugs could heal him. His generation believed doctors knew best, and a pill could fix things. It was propaganda. He was brainwashed into thinking all he needed were specific pills to live, and he didn't need to change his lifestyle. When he retired, he indulged in rich food coupled with daily drinking. His attitude was he had earned the right to live like a king. Which led to a slow and painful death.

Rejecting food altogether isn't the answer, though. My late trainer Jennifer was part of the women's first body-building circuit. She was my fitness guru. I was in awe of her ability to maintain a low body fat percentage. She was a pioneer in the bodybuilding field who broke down barriers for women. What you didn't see were her low self-esteem and poor self-worth. She was never satisfied with the way she looked, and she was a constant project, working on herself. I'm pretty sure she had undiagnosed body dysmorphia. She was consumed with her hamstrings, shoulder, or when her next therapy session was. She always tried the latest treatments—laser therapy, hot and cold therapy, injections of PRP, and many other therapies and supplements. She lived in the gym, and she lost faith in nutrition and lived almost primarily on supplements. Once, I saw her take a handful of thirty pills, and I gasped. She said, "I take these three times a day." She was mostly living on supplements, always telling herself that if she fixed her body, then the rest of her life would turn out. One day, she didn't wake up. Her heart stopped, and her body shut down. It was a form of anorexia. I was stunned how this *health professional* who looked so lean and svelte on the outside was dying on the inside. She was slowly killing herself by lifestyle disease.

Food is here for our enjoyment and to bring us nourishment. God made food the way he intended us to eat it. Processing the food is what adds in the bad things the body cannot process, so it stores it as fat or irregular cells. The best way to nourish the body is to eat less-processed food. Whole foods with water and fiber fill you up and keep your energy and blood sugar levels stable.

There is nothing new, except what has been forgotten.

—Marie Antoinette

FASTING

Our bodies heal themselves. When someone is sick, they go to the doctor. But a doctor is nothing more than a licensed drug dealer. You pay the co-pay and leave with a prescription.

When my mom was sick, she stopped everything and resigned herself to bed. I never understood why she didn't run to the doctor's office like most people normally do. She was essentially fasting to allow her body to heal itself. Fasting is a time-tested, ancient tradition. It has been used not only for weight loss but to improve concentration, extend life, prevent insulin resistance, and even reverse the aging process.

Fasting has been around for thousands of years. It can be spiritual, religious, medical, or to break an addiction. Think of your digestive organs as your employees, working for you to produce energy and clear thinking. If you never gave your employees a day off, how could they function optimally? So, I like to fast on Mondays. I drink lots of water and give my digestion a rest and a chance to catch up. When I resume eating on Tuesday, I stick closely to plant based foods. Here are some of my favorite quick and easy recipes.

PLANT BASED RECIPES

Stir-fry Vegetables
1 head of cabbage
1 bunch of broccolis
1 cup - whole cashews
1 pint - vegetable broth
Braggs Amino Acids to taste
Ginger
Garlic

Cut up the broccoli, grate the ginger and garlic, and simmer in the vegetable broth for ten minutes until tender. Add in the chopped-up cabbage. Place lid on pot, and simmer for another ten minutes, then add the cashews and amino acids. Let stand for ten minutes with no heat—portion into jars.

Kale Chips
1 - bunch of fresh kale
Pink Himalayan Salt
½ tsp olive oil

Devein the kale and wash. Pat dry, and tear into bite-sized pieces. Lightly spray the baking sheet. Lay the dry kale on the metal baking sheet, toss with 1 tsp of olive oil, and grind salt over the top. Lightly toss again, broil on high for five minutes, lightly toss and broil for another five mins. Using broil on high leave the oven slightly cracked open.

Sweet Potatoes
4-6 large sweet potatoes
Garlic powder
Pink Himalayan salt
1 tsp Olive oil

Skin the potatoes with a vegetable peeler and chop into small cubes. Toss with salt and oil, bake at 350 degrees for thirty minutes, then broil for five minutes.

Potato Skin Chips
Sweet potato skins (from previous recipe)
Salt

Chop sweet potato skins into bite-size pieces. Spread out on cookie sheet. Sprinkle with salt. Broil for five minutes. Lightly toss, and broil five more minutes.

Broccoli Parmesan
One bunch of broccolis
Parmesan cheese grated
Oil

Cut broccoli into bite-size pieces, wash, lay on cookie sheet, toss with oil, and generously cover with parmesan. Bake at 350 degrees for twenty minutes, until desired tenderness.

Sweet Peppers filled with Taco flavored Cauliflower Rice
4-6 large sweet peppers, all colors
Cauliflower, one large bunch
Taco seasoning package
Mushrooms
Asparagus
Grated parmesan cheese

Cut sweet peppers in half and remove the seeds and white part (veins). Cut so they will stand alone like a bowl. Wash and set aside. Chop up cauliflower and season with taco spices or a package of taco seasoning—mix in chopped up mushrooms, and asparagus. Fill the peppers with the mixture and top with parmesan cheese. Bake at 350 degrees for thirty-five minutes.

Green Smoothie
1 cup of kale
1 cucumber—peeled and cut up
1 honey crisp apple (remove the seeds)
2 mint leaves
10 almonds
Squeeze of lemon
The juice of one orange
2 cups of water

Add everything to the blender for sixty seconds, stir, and blend again for sixty more seconds.

Red Smoothie
1 cup of strawberries
½ cup raspberries
1 cup water
½ cup oatmeal
½ cup unsweetened almond milk
½ banana
Agave to taste

Blend for sixty seconds.

Chocolate Covered Strawberries
Wash and dry ripened strawberries
1 cup 80% dark chocolate

Melt chocolate in a double boiler, dip strawberries in melted chocolate, place on parchment paper, refrigerate for ten minutes, then enjoy. Eat within two days.

Energy Balls
12 dates pitted
¼ tsp cocoa
½ cup raw almonds
½ cup cashews
½ cup water
Honey to taste

Place all the ingredients in the blender. Blend until mixture is sticky. On wax paper, roll into 1-inch balls and refrigerate in an airtight container.

Staples Prepped in the frig ready to grab.
Cucumbers, peel and slice.
Carrots, peel and cut into spears.
Cherry tomatoes
Celery wash cut into spears
Iceberg lettuce
Bib lettuce
Romain lettuce
Kale
Almonds
Cashews
Apples
Oranges
Grapes
Peaches
Watermelon

Having these foods prepped and ready makes for a great week. I can *grab* whatever I need *and go*. When I eat, it's either because I am hungry, or I want to maintain a healthy weight. I am not puffy anymore, and the layer of fat has melted off of my hips and legs. There is no more chaos around food. It's so liberating, finally. I can enjoy life, eat, and be healthy. You can, too. For more recipes, go to my website, www.crystalwaltman.com or, share with me your favorite plant-based snacks or meals.

CHAPTER 9

QUIT RUNNING SOMEONE ELSE'S RACE

BACK TALK

Every set back is a set up for a greater come back. God wants to bring you out better than you were before.

—Joel Osteen

Whe I woke up, I was lying on the floor, staring up at the ceiling. I didn't know how I had gotten there or how much time had passed, but I felt the dry tears on my cheeks. *Where am I?* I scanned the room. *Why am I on the floor in the closet?* I tried to get up, but my body wouldn't respond. My legs wouldn't move. So, I army-crawled out of the closet and across the cold tile floor of the bathroom, about twenty yards. I pulled myself up to the bed and reached for the phone. I wasn't crying, but I felt tears running down my face. *What is happening?* I thought. I had no control over my lower body, so I called my husband and asked him to pick up our daughter from school. Exhausted from the effort, I soon dozed off.

I woke up to the voice of my daughter. "Mommy?" I opened my eyes, and tears flooded my vision. My arms reach out for a hug to reassure her. "Everything will be okay." I didn't even believe this myself.

———⟨∞⟩———

My first memory of back pain was at the age of eighteen after a weekend softball tournament in college. My roommate and I were hostages to the couch in our dorm room, so the party came to us as we sat in our inflammation. She was the pitcher, and I played first base. We shared many first-time experiences in college—like the dryness of going through Accutane. We were sore and peeling because of a waxing experience turned into a disaster after we could not get the wax off.

We were soldiers in our sport. Our bodies were inflamed, and our backs were screaming. We left it all on the field and iced on and off. The pain was debilitating in the days following a tournament. We numbed it with alcohol, extra-strength ibuprofen, ice, and any cream we could get our hands on.

I continued to live with back pain after college. I thought if I stopped playing and took up yoga, I could heal myself. So, I pursued a spine specialist's opinion, and they said I was missing two discs. They recommended surgery, but I didn't want surgery. I was in denial that at twenty years old, I was physically broken. Though I tried all kinds of natural pain management, including chiropractic, cold therapy, cupping, acupuncture, Thai massages, and yoga, the relief they provided was short-lived. I put the blame back on myself: *If only I lost weight, I would be in less pain.* So, I continued to practice yoga routinely and drank for pain management.

Although the pain had been going on for almost twenty years, I enjoyed spending more time outdoors as my physically sober life continued to evolve. I enjoyed all of it, but the pain that was once slightly tolerable started to come back after any activity. Because of my new commitment to sobriety, I could no longer carelessly self-medicate and numb the pain with oxycodone or even think about using pills. Life seemed to be going very well, but everyday activities like going to the mall or sitting in a theater had slowly become extremely difficult. Instead of spending the day in bed due to a hangover, I now spent the day in bed because of back pain.

I wish I had a great story to tell you about how I broke my back, like running from a bear while hiking before I fell off a cliff to save my life. But that never happened. When we bought a new house, I was ecstatic! The adrenaline was pumping through my veins. It was a natural high of life's positive stressors. You're asking yourself, *did the house break your back?* We had the help of movers for the first few days, but I don't think I sat down for two weeks. I was determined to put everything in its place—it was what a new homeowner should do, after all. After I unpacked all the boxes, our routine resumed at the new location. A few days later, I was doing laundry, humming with joy as I walked into my new master closet. This closet was beautiful, one I had only dreamed of. Now I had a *side*—I didn't have to squish my clothes into my share of the small closet (made even smaller by its rolling mirror doors). In the old house, I gave up most of the closet space to my husband because I was not working at the time and wore mostly yoga clothes or jeans. I was buzzing through the new house on laundry day, and I lifted the basket of clothes out of my new fancy built-in hamper and *pow*! It felt like a blistering bullet had just ripped into my back.

The next day, I needed help sitting up and walking. When I got up, my left foot turned out, and my left leg was dragging. Pain shot down the backside of my leg, deep in my glutes, down to the foot. I was terrified because I had never felt pain like that before. My husband took me to see three different doctors to see what had happened.

My disc had fully blown up. I had a massive herniated disc, missing discs, and a broken back in two places. The doctors compared my broken back to a gymnast or lineman's broken body. My laundry basket was literally the straw that broke the camel's back. They found that my bones were not holding me up—my core muscular system was.

The diagnosis was conclusive, but the treatments were all different.

Even though I was dying in pain, my instincts told me that the first two doctors weren't right for me. They talked about how awful my life was going to be, and the word *recovery* was only a word. My goal, even in that moment of intense pain, was to recover and get back to the active lifestyle I loved so much. After all, I had a five-year-old daughter who needed me more than anyone I ever knew, and not playing an active role in her life was unthinkable.

My third consultation was with Dr. Salari. He was young compared to the other consultations, and he was what you wanted in a surgeon—kind, compassionate, soft-spoken, and positive. Primarily working with athletes, he had seen others return to their sports successfully. He was optimistic and wanted to do the most surgery, not the least.

He said, "If we just do the discectomy, the other part of your back will fail you sooner than later. You'll be back on the table in a year or two." After he consulted with several colleagues, he called me. He said, "I have a plan. I will redo the entire L3, L4, L5, S1 and discectomy." He went on to explain he had not done this much surgery on one person before, and it would not be easy, but if I was up for it, so was he.

I agreed to a two-part, seven-hour surgery.

Three days later, I was in a seven-hour surgery. I was scared for several reasons. Because I had witnessed bad stories of pain-pill addiction, I was terrified because of my history with addiction. Second, would I ever walk properly again, much less be able to run?

The doctor cut in three places, one on each side of the spine to make room for a cage made from two eight-inch rods, eight screws, and three new discs. He stitched me up, then turned me over on my side for a final cut right above the side hip bone for the discectomy. (A discectomy is the removal of massively bulging damaged discs.)

After the surgery, I stayed in the hospital for a week. My family and friends visited and helped me walk a few steps every day. I could hardly make it out of my room when I left the hospital. It was so painful to get up.

RECOVERING FROM BACK SURGERY

Along with regular visits with Dr. Salari, I also worked closely with my naturopathic doctor to manage the pain and the drugs that came with it. Dr. Salari said, "Don't bend, twist, or lift for three months!" My surgery was different than a knee replacement surgery, where they want you to start bending it right away. I spent six weeks in a back brace, and the healing was excruciating. Taking as little pain medication as I could, I waited for the pain to return and really take hold before I swallowed another pill. I took them sparingly for approximately two weeks, and followed recovery protocol.

I became a master at the steamroll. With a flat back and brace on, I swayed back and forth to get some momentum to roll to the side, and push my body up with my arms.

Walking was a chore. My body said, *Stay in bed; you need the rest.* I fought the thought and got up every day and walked until I was exhausted. Some days, it was only for five minutes. For six months, I couldn't even do simple tasks like making a bed or loading the dishwasher. I started physical therapy three months after surgery and worked through the pain three times a week.

Recovering from back surgery seemed impossible on most days, and to this day, it is one of the toughest things I've ever done. Compared to giving birth, this was harder and lasted a bit longer.

LIFE AFTER BACK SURGERY

> What if pain—like love—
> is just a place brave people visit?

—Glennon Doyle Melton,
Love Warrior

I was petrified I wouldn't be able to walk again. This was a deeply humbling experience. However, three years post-surgery, I have no pain! Dr. Salari is a magician. I can walk and move like a normal person, and I continue to practice yoga a minimum of twice a week as part of my *ingredients for life*. I do not do any deep twists—my yoga practice is about only 80% of any class. I don't judge myself or compare myself to others. You know—don't run someone else's race. Before the rods, I was very flexible. Now, my flexibility is average, but that's all right. Now, I know more than ever the importance of walking and staying flexible. I walk a lot, and I hike. If I had known how liberating it is to be out of physical pain, I would have had the surgery a long time ago.

Dr. Salari, of DISC (Desert Institute of Spine Care), credits my successful recovery to going into surgery healthy and at an ideal body weight. This was the longest, most intense surgery he had ever performed. Because I embodied the will to recover, I now have a better life than I did before. I will never take for granted the little things in life, like showering, picking toys up off the floor, or making a bed. I am blessed daily, and I can enjoy each day pain-free.

My perspective on health and competing has shifted. I would tell my younger self to listen to her body, and that it's not about "no pain, no gain."

The Link between Alcohol and Osteoporosis

Alcohol negatively affects bone health for several reasons. To begin with, excessive alcohol interferes with the balance of calcium, an essential nutrient for healthy bones. Calcium balance may be further disrupted by alcohol's ability to interfere with the production of vitamin D, a vitamin essential for calcium absorption.

In addition, chronic heavy drinking can cause hormone deficiencies in men and women. Men with alcoholism may produce less testosterone, a hormone linked to the production of osteoblasts (the cells that stimulate bone formation). In women, chronic alcohol exposure can trigger irregular menstrual cycles, a factor that reduces estrogen levels, increasing the risk for osteoporosis. Also, cortisol levels may be elevated in people with alcoholism. Cortisol is known to decrease bone formation and increase bone breakdown.

Because of the effects of alcohol on balance and gait, people with alcoholism tend to fall more frequently than those without the disorder. Heavy alcohol consumption has been linked to an increase in the risk of fracture, including the most serious kind—hip fracture. Vertebral fractures are also more common in chronic heavy drinkers.

(To read the full article, go to https://www.bones.nih.gov/health-info/bones/osteoporosis/conditions-behaviors/alcoholism)

Deep down, I believe I got into health and fitness because I tended to be *thick*, as I heard in high school. I studied nutrition and food, how to manipulate overeating and drinking, and keeping an ideal body weight.

My mother was a nondrinker and stressed: *Alcohol has so many calories.* "If he would just cut out the booze ..." she mused, referring to my stepdad and his growing waistline. That recording played over and over in my head and led to alcoholic bulimia. I would have rather drank than ate. I wanted to get the buzz quicker—who would want to delay with food? Either way, I didn't want the calories. When my stomach was full of booze, I threw up and kept drinking. The next day I weighted my dehydrated-self and nodded with approval. "Okay, I did not gain any weight." No matter what state I was in the next day, I worked out and showed up for practice. And as long as I showed up for the workout, nobody ever thought there was a problem. That allowed me to detox to *re-tox*, a motto I used to go by that now makes me empathetic when I overhear people at the gym talk about the drunken night they're now sweating out.

The most profound lesson that came out of the back surgery was learning to feel comfortable in my skin. I love all my scars as they are part of the road map of my life. I only have one body. I have learned to love the one I've got.

HOW TO KEEP A HEALTHY BACK

Limit impact—this wears out your discs.
Stay flexible—the hamstrings will pull on the back and create pain if they are tight. Bending over to touch your toes is an easy daily release.
Roll—have a roller at home to work the calf and hamstrings.
Walk—movement will keep everything loose. Try for 7,000 steps a day.
Maintain a strong core—a strong core really helps support the spine.

As a trainer for two decades, I worked with many clients who had back disease, mostly due to an imbalance in the body. I would stretch clients before and after their workout and encourage a recovery routine, like yoga, swimming pool walking, water aerobics or using a kick board. I taught high-impact classes, too, and ran for years, both on the treadmill and outside. Now with new cardio technology, you can achieve the same result without high impact on the body and save yourself the wear and tear.

MORNING STRETCH ROUTINE

Daily Breathing

Face the mirror with your feet together, pointed straight in front of you. Put your heels together, toes touching. Ridiculously easy as this seems, you might find it hard. Your toes will want to spread themselves out for balance, but don't let them. Keep them together, and soon enough, you won't feel as if your about to fall to one side.

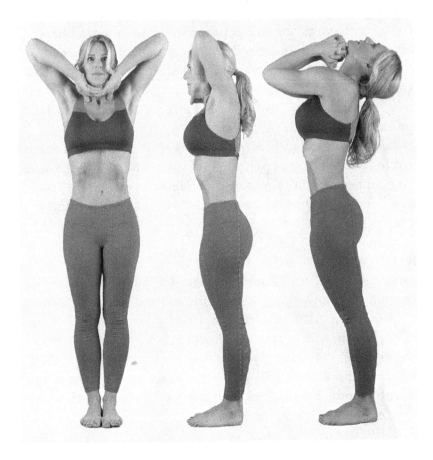

Place your hands together and interlace the knuckles, touching the underside of the chin. The elbows are together, and the thumbs are touching the throat. Maintain this contact throughout the exercise.

Inhale deeply through the nose, mouth closed, for a slow count of six. Fill up those lungs! At the same time, slowly raise your elbows like seagull wings on either side of your head. Lower your chin downward onto the knuckles, the very center of your two wings. Don't bend forward—just lower your chin. When you've inhaled completely and reached the count of six, drop your head back as far as it can go, keeping your mouth open halfway while slowly and steadily exhaling for another count of six. As you do that, bring your forearms, elbows, and wrists together in front of your face. Keep your chin in firm contact with your knuckles. Force out every last bit of air. Your upturned face and the length of your arms form one straight even line from the wall behind you to the mirror in front of you.

Do ten of these inhale-exhale cycles. At the end of the final exhale, bring your head back to an upright position, let your arms fall naturally to your side, and rest a moment. Then, raise arms again to interlock the hand and begin again.

You may feel slightly dizzy as you do this because you're not used to so much oxygen pouring into your system! The dizziness will disappear as you gain more experience. Keep your eyes open the whole time. Otherwise, you may lose your balance and fall over.

Benefits

Standing Deep Breathing uses up to one hundred percent of your lung capacity to get the stale air out and avoid respiratory problems, such as bronchitis, emphysema, asthma, and shortness of breath. It also teaches us how to sustain your inhales and exhales rather than gasp. By expanding the lungs, Standing Deep Breathing stimulates circulation, so it wakes up the muscles and the entire body. For that reason, it is a good warm-up before any other kind of exercise.

Half Moon

Stand with your feet together, raise your arms over your head, and bring your hands together, interlocking the fingers into a nice tight grip. Release the index finger, straighten and press them together. They're going to be pointed to the top of the church steeple you'll form with your head and arms. Raise and straighten your arms completely on either side of your head, interlock in the elbows. Reach upward, strongly pressure your arms against your ears. Keep your head and chin up, looking forward.

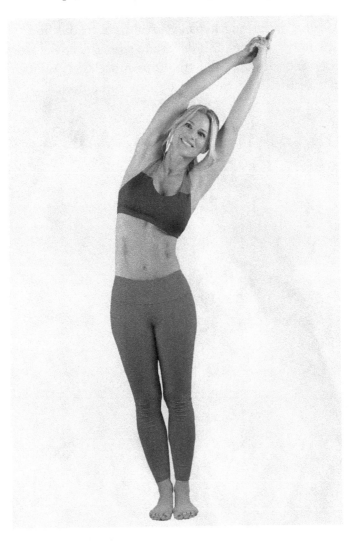

Push your hips to the left, and without flexing your arms or legs, slowly bend your right side as much as possible. Keep the whole-body facing front. Keep your arms straight, elbows locked, and don't let your chin sink into your chest—keep it three inches away. As you stretch your upper body to the right, continue to push both hips directly to the left—feel the beautiful pull along the left side of the body. (Now you can look in the mirror, and you'll see why we called this half-moon) Repeat on the other side.

Benefits

Half Moon Pose strengthens every muscle in the body's core, especially in the abdomen. It flexes and strengthens the latissimus dorsi, oblique, deltoid, and trapezius muscles. It increases the flexibility of the spine from the coccyx to the neck.

Hands to Feet

It would seem like bending over touching your toes is easy, but it is not. It is a use it or lose it movement. The reason I show this variation because it is as far as I can go post back surgery, and it is OK. I am not running anyone else's race.

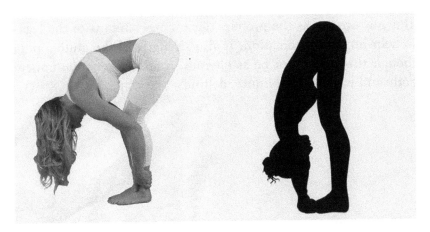

With your feet together nicely, as in half moon, lift the torso, then bend forward from the hips, legs straight, stretching and reaching as far down as you can go. When you can no longer keep your legs straight, bend the knees, and reach back and take hold of your heels with your hands, thumbs and four fingers touching the floor. Bend your elbows, and press the inside of your forearm completely against the back of your calves. The goal is to touch your elbows together behind your legs eventually.

Stretch your body as much as possible toward the floor. Try to lay your stomach on top of your thighs. Place your chest on your knees so there are no gaps visible from the side. Your face is against your legs somewhere below the knees, and eyes are wide open.

Now, slowly push your knees back, keep your upper and lower body glued together, and straighten your legs as much as possible. Your weight should be forward on your toes. Put your weight on your heels, and lift your hips towards the ceiling. Leg straight! Lock your knees! Try harder! This kind of pain is normal, expected, and good.

Hold for a count of ten, and breathe normally, then let go of the heels and come up slowly and gracefully.

Benefits

This posture works the muscles, ligaments, tendons of the legs to help improve circulation. It also strengthens the glutes, and though this might not be as obvious, it strengthens the upper body and back—the obliques, deltoids, and trapezius.

Back Bend

Open up your heart (yes literally). Bending back allows you to open up and not feel stuck.

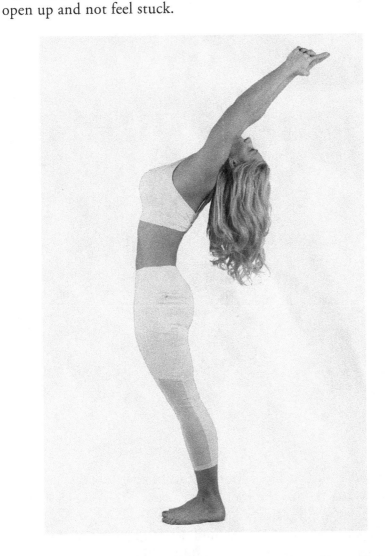

Put your arms overhead, your palms together, elbows locked, hands together, and push the hips forward. Drop your arms back and open up the chest. Mouth closed and breath normal.

Awkward Pose
Work your leg and concentration without doing a sled press or going to the gym.

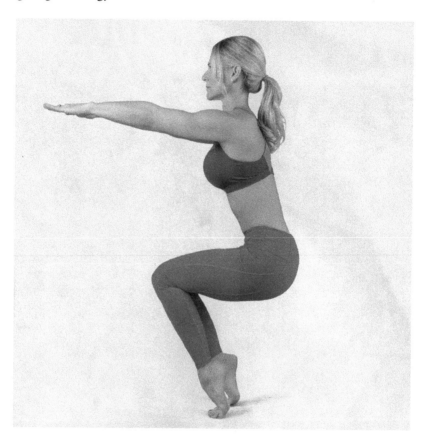

Stand with you feet about six inches apart, or the space of both fists together on the floor between your feet. Raise your arms straight out in front of you, parallel with the floor, palms down and fingers together. There should be about six inches between your two arms, and the rest should be about six inches apart. Don't let your arm muscles go slack, keep them nice and tight.

With your heels flat on the floor, exhale completely, and sit down as deeply as you can as if you are sitting in an imaginary chair behind you until your thighs are parallel to the floor. (If you can't sit down deep enough to bring your thighs parallel at first, don't be concerned. Only the very limber among you will be able to do this at first.)

While keeping your weight in your heels, lift your chest, and lean your upper body backward while stretching your fingertips forward towards the mirror in front of you. Keep six inches of the space between the toes, heels, knees, and hands. Count to ten slowly.

Benefits

Awkward Pose will tone and shape your legs like nobody's business. Plus, the definition and strength you gain here are among some of the fastest results. This is such a great warm-up in part because it stimulates circulation, sending blood roaring to the lower extremities. If you suffer from chronically cold feet, that will be over. It will also help relieve rheumatism and arthritis in the legs and help to cure slipped discs and other problems in the lower spine. Awkward Pose also promotes laser-beam concentration.

Push Ups

Push-Ups The push-up goes back to the late, great Jack Lalanne. He introduced the push-up to the mainstream and proposed working out with only body weight. He made the push-up popular for setting a record in 1956 for the most push-ups.

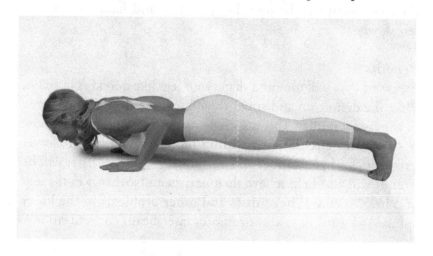

In the plank position, keep your wrist, hands, and shoulders parallel, and hold belly button in tight. Lower yourself to the ground, and push yourself back up to a plank.

Benefits

Push-ups strengthens the chest, triceps, balance and posture by focusing on a strong core. Repeat 10 times.

Down Dog
This posture probably gets more jokes than any other pose. It is the first thing someone will say after you say the word, "yoga." This posture is hard, and I love it for the calf-stretching.

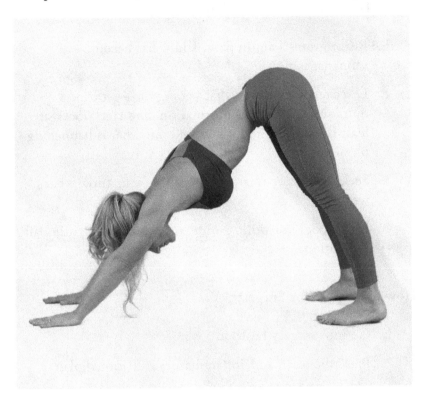

With hands and palms on the floor, hips pointing to the air, spine straight, heels touching the mat, legs only hip-distance apart; tilt hips to the sky, and flatten back. Keep head aligned with the spine. Inhale through the nose, and exhale with mouth open, like lions' breath.

Benefits
Stretches the shoulder, hamstrings, calves, arches, hands, arms, and legs. It gets the blood flowing to your head and makes you feel energized.

I love walking in the pool in the morning. The cold, fresh water and air reduce inflammation, and I also pool walk and swim with a kickboard several laps for about ten minutes.

If you Have Back Pain Get Help

1. Realization - I am in pain, and it has become unmanageable.

2. Discovery - Evaluate what's going on—get expert opinions, gather test information, and facts. Seek at least three consultations to find out what is happening physiologically.

3. Seek alternative treatment now that you know what's wrong.

4. If this does not work, go for surgery after weighting all the options.

How to Prepare for Surgery

1. Go into surgery healthy.

2. Prescribe to an anti-inflammatory nutritional plan.

3. Be at your ideal body weight.

4. Have a recovery plan and a team to help you overcome the side effects of pills (including depression, constipation, etc.).

5. Walk every day, no matter what.

6. Drink plenty of water.

When you get out of emotional and physical pain, you can live a life unencumbered. A life of choice is exciting. You do not have to live with back pain. Find out what's going on and find a way to make peace with it. Look for a support group in your area. There is a thriving class at my health club called, "Happy Back." At any time, everyone is at some stage of the process with their back pain. For more discussion on Back Talk, go to CrystalWaltman.com and share your story. We got your back.

CHAPTER 10
QUIT TURNING OFF YOUR INNER VOICE

LIFE SKILLS LEARNED FROM SOFTBALL

Hard work beats talent when talent doesn't work hard.

—Tom Notke

I zipped up my softball bag over twenty years ago, and I just recently unzipped it two-plus decades later when my daughter asked me if she could play softball. When I unzipped it, I contemplated all the dirt, sweat, and bruises from my years playing the sport. My daughter, now nine-years-old, helped me pull the heavy black vinyl bat bag down from the attic. The bag had been stored at my mom's house for many years until we bought a house, and she said, "It's time to come get your stuff—we are moving out and downsizing." So, I picked up my sporting equipment, yearbooks, and trophies. On the drive home, I'd looked at the bag in silence with flashbacks of pain, not knowing if I would ever unzip it.

It had been twenty-one years since the last time I played. When I opened the bag, I pulled out the equipment piece by piece—holding each one up to my nose and smelling it, touching it, feeling the dry, crispy leather of the gloves on my hand. I shared stories with my daughter of all the joy the sport had brought me. Being part of a competitive club team gave me connections all over the world. At a young age I realized there was a different way to live. I used to hear—*we can't afford it* from my parents. But once I played for a while and spent time with other families, I noticed a common theme. They would ask—*how can we afford it?* Then I was given the book by Robert Kiyosaki which explains this concept well, "Rich Dad Poor Dad."

A teammate's dad was in the lemonade business—specifically, he was a vendor for sporting stadi-

HOW CAN WE AFFORD IT?

ums. He allowed the girls on the team to work by selling lemonade at baseball games to make money to help unburden their parents for the cost of equipment, travel fees, etc. This was a game-changer for me because it gave me the opportunity to make money when I needed to and to learn how to work smarter, not harder.

The bat bag would not unzip because the zipper was rotted, so we had to cut it open with a pair of scissors. It reminded me of what it was like to be a part of something bigger than myself. There were two first basemen's gloves, a regular fielding glove, and two bats inside of the bag. I pulled out a thirty-year-old glove, tapped if off, and as I did, the leftover dirt from all those years ago imploded in my face. The smell of the dirt brought back so many memories. There was a dirty sock, sunflower seeds, and a bottle of grape Gatorade. Liv and I smiled as I grabbed the ball and popped it into the glove. To hear the pop of the glove again was almost surreal. It took me many years to process the bad memories associated with the sport and to have a spiritual enlightenment. But I reached the point I could pass on positive values and character traits I picked up from the sport.

I played competitively from the ages of ten to twenty with over 3,000 games of softball and more than 10,000 hours of practice. I will share with you the ritual of sport I mastered.

Through the sport, I learned about preparation, visualization, time, team, and commitment.

PREPARATION

The night before the game, my jersey (#33, sometimes #13) hung over my desk chair. I polished my cleats and opened the bat bag to ensure everything was in the right place—glove, batting gloves, ball, bat, sunflower seeds, tape, extra hair tie, cleats (freshly polished), socks, and contact solution. I laid my pants next to my jersey and placed my warmup shoes on the floor with my long socks delicately folded over. I got my water jug out and placed it by the sink. Then, I drank some water, ate a balanced meal, and prepared for sleep.

The bat bag would not unzip because the zipper was rotted. We ended up having to cut it open with a pair of scissors. It reminded me of what it was like to be a part of something bigger than myself. There were two first basemen's gloves, a regular fielding glove, and two bats inside of the bag. I pulled out the thirty-year-old glove, slapped it with my other hand and the leftover dirt from all those years ago imploded in my face. The smell of the dirt brought back so many memories. There was a dirty sock, a bag of sunflower seeds, and a bottle of half empty expired grape Gatorade. Liv and I smiled as I grabbed the ball and began tossing it into the glove. This is mind-blowing to think it through: *You mean if I show up on time, prepare, and play like I practice, I will win?* Yes, sports and life are that simple—you can out-hustle your opponent through preparation, visualization, time, team, and commitment. Even if your opponent was born with more natural talent, you can out-train them. If I do the same thing over and over, I can surpass someone who has natural talent.

When you show up prepared on the field and in life, you are already ahead of 90% of the people who go through life unconscious of their surroundings. There are three types of people.

The *Pulled-It-Off Patty* says, "I pulled it off! I am here on time—wait, what time *is* it? — but anyway, I'm here. I made it."

Then, she takes a breath. "I might be missing something, but I know it's in there somewhere." Second is *Scattered Sally*, always running late, always so busy, and always a tornado when she arrives. She unloads her problems on the team when she arrives. And lastly, there's the *Peaceful Warrior*. She is early, because early is on-time, on-time is late, and late is unacceptable. She is prepared and calm, knows where everything is, and she knows the opponent.

> EARLY IS ON-TIME, ON-TIME IS LATE, AND LATE IS UNACCEPTABLE

Softball taught me unwavering preparation. If you fail to plan, you plan to fail. The alcoholic *thinking problem* of repetitive thoughts is beneficial if you apply it to sports or to everyday life. Now, I get so much joy out of watching my daughter finish homework, zip her school bag up with everything in it, place her lunch box and water bottle by the sink, and set out her clothes for the next day. Then, she takes a bath and relaxes. Because of her preparation, our mornings are great. I feel like the luckiest parent on earth because the mornings are our happy time. We sit together and connect after she gets up, makes her bed, combs her hair, and feeds the dog. When she's done with her morning routine, she pulls a stool up to the breakfast bar and says, "Good morning, Mom, I slept great!" *It's a Beautiful Day, by* U2 is playing in the background. *It's a beautiful day, don't let it slip away.* I see the spirit of the peaceful warrior in her, and it makes my heart smile.

VISUALIZATION

Visualization is daydreaming with a purpose. I step into the batter's box and twist the dirt with the right ball of my foot, as if

> VISUALIZATION IS DAYDREAMING WITH A PURPOSE

I was squashing a bug. The outfielder starts taking steps backwards. I root my body in the batter's box outlined with white chalk, and I gently double tap the home plate with my bat.

Raising the bat to my shoulder, I wiggle my fingers, bend my knees, take a deep breath, grip the bat, look at the pitcher, and everything goes silent as I wait for the perfect pitch. I am prepared for this moment.

Do you try on your clothes the day before? Do you visualize yourself completing the next task you have to complete? These were habits I picked up in high school. We didn't have uniforms, so the night before school I liked to try on a few outfits to see which one felt the best for the following day. My favorite day was Friday's during football season. We wore our cheerleading uniforms to school for the pep rallies. I was always glad to wear a sports uniform. The material is prepared for action, the cuts are purposeful and performance-ready. By wearing a uniform, you are part of something bigger.

When I was on the bench watching the other team approach the field, I visualized myself hitting a long ball, running around the bases, and crossing home plate. My team was lined up for high fives and congratulated me on my home run and RBI's (runs batted in).

Then, I pictured myself making the play at first base and whipped the ball around in a star position. I could hear the snap of the ball in each glove, and I could see my catcher whizzing the ball to me after a strikeout and holding up her pointer finger and pinkie, yelling, "Two down!" I could also picture the coach's face after the game and hear his praise, "Great game, girls."

Sometimes, when we won, our coach was upset because we had made too many errors. In sports class, we studied footage of the pitcher we'd face at the next game. All week, I'd watch the tapes and visualize hitting against this pitcher. When I visualized myself hitting and running around the bases, I felt a sense of belonging: *I have been here before, and this is exactly where I am supposed to be.* I visualized this over and over in my head. Do you have a visual image of yourself completing the next task on your to-do list?

Some people think positive visualization is a substitute for faith. They are two different things. Faith is giving your life over to God and knowing where you're going in the afterlife. Visualization is a skill you have to practice to hone. It can be simple or complex, but it is as straightforward as seeing a mental image in your head.

I decided to write this book at the age of forty. It took me two years to pull the trigger and get started, and two years to get over my mental minefields. One of the first things my publisher told me to do was to make an, "I am an author" video. This guy spoke my language! I understood this exercise because of the visualization techniques I used in sports. You have to see it in your head to make it happen. I don't consider myself a *writer*, but I am fortunate to add author to my toolbox of life and can leave this book as part of my legacy.

TIME

I like the acronym TIME, which stands for Things I Must Earn. When I was in high school, the *no pass no play* rule was enforced. My choice was simple—do my homework so I could do the thing I loved. I did not love schoolwork or studying, but I didn't hate it either. It was a currency to get what I wanted. If I got good grades, I could play sports and be part of a team. I yearned for belonging. Academics was a straightforward time-management issue, a building block, a step stool, and then a ladder to what I wanted. Success can come from what you don't do. As Joel Osteen says, "You can't hang out with chickens and expect to soar with the eagles." How you spend your time is a direct reflection of what you believe is important. I spent time preparing the night before. I even took study hall to free up time after school. When you practice something over and over again, it becomes easier and mindless. This includes homework and time spent in the batting cage. You want muscle memory to kick in on the days you are tired or the days you don't really want to do it. Your body will do the next right thing because you have built your habits to reflect your priorities.

COMMITMENT

The beginning and the end—the seasons of sports reflect it. To know there is a beginning and end of a season is refreshing. It makes it easy to digest the commitment—*Well, I can do this for nine months (or a weekend, or a season, or a tournament)*. When you break life down into small milestones, it becomes very manageable, and it can be so much fun.

I am in the season of raising school-age kiddos. So, my life revolves around the school schedule, which, fortunately, makes it very simple to plan and achieve milestones. The first quarter is nine weeks until fall when there is a one-week break. The second quarter is nine weeks followed by two weeks off for Christmas break. The third quarter is nine weeks long followed by a one-week spring break. The fourth quarter is nine weeks followed by summer break, which is twelve weeks long. Principles of time management and commitment are things I learned in sports and translate to everyday life. Each season seems very doable and enjoyable when broken down in small increments.

Time is an intangible thing. If you have ever spent time with a dying person, you may have heard them say, "I wish I would have spent more time with so-and-so and less time working and more time doing such-and-such." In her book, *Parent on Purpose*, Amy Carney writes about a penny jar. She understands her time as a parent is limited, so she wants to spend it with purpose and without regret. So, she suggests having two jars, one to calculate how many weeks are left until your kid turns eighteen, and then put that number of pennies in the first jar. Every Sunday, you move one penny to the other jar. This is how she visualized time and revitalized her commitment as a parent.

TEAM

Being a part of a team is having an extended family for a season. If you make the cut, you are sisters for a season. We may not have known each other before, but we are brought together by a common goal, and we will forever be bonded over it. We will have wins and losses, and we will see this through together.

Team sports tend to give women and girls the things they otherwise have a hard time getting like resilience, grit, knowledge of teamwork, and knowledge of leadership. All of these things are crucial, and they all are learned probably better on a sports team than anywhere else," said Debora Spar, a professor at Harvard Business School, who moderated a panel about women in sports, leadership, and empowerment that the school hosted on campus earlier this year.

In general, I like people, especially women, but sometimes you meet a girl who's peanut butter and jealous. She either wants to be you or wants to wear your skin. It is hard to tell which (and sometimes, it's both). After I left my parents' house at age eighteen, I had many roommates both in college and after. During college, one of my roommates was a jealous redheaded tomboyish homebody who got jealous whenever I left the dorm. One time, she went so far as to let the air out of my bike tires to keep me from leaving! Yet, when I stayed at home, she wouldn't spend time with me. She enjoyed her Cheetos and coke while watching TV—making sure the TV faced only toward her side of the room. At the time, I was shocked by this, but it prepared me for what was to come in real life.

Playing team sports prepares you by learning how to deal with different personalities. When you apply this experience in adult life or the workforce, you either see people as opponents or teammates.

Here are some of my favorite quotes about the values I learned from softball:

Life Is Not Measured by the Number of Breaths
We Take, but by the Moments That Take Our Breath Away.
— Unknown Author.

Frank Lloyd Wright, a 20th Century American architect once said, "No Stream rises higher than its source." His reference to "source" means *you*.

MANAGING TIME IN THE REAL WORLD

This simple concept was hard for me to learn, but once I honed this skill, it was a game changer. There are some who put fires out all day and that's the way they operate. In our house, my husband refers to it as—*slay the dragons*. He does a great job at it. I operate from a place of peace, purpose, and preparation. Your lack of preparation is not my emergency. When I compartmentalize my time, things can get done to my satisfaction. I hardly ever say things like—*I pulled it off anymore*. When I hear people say this, it makes me cringe and feel pity for everyone involved.

A WEEK IN MY LIFE

I take my work-from-home-CPO (Chief Parenting Officer) role very seriously. Though I am purposeful about my time with my daughter, I'm also intentional about what I do when I'm *not* with her. I return home from school drop off at 8:00 a.m., and I have until 2:00 p.m. for school pick-up. This allows me six hours a day, five days a week, or thirty hours a week.

To run my house, I have four loads of laundry. Monday's are my house day, which is when I spend the day completing all my house-related work. I decline any invitations on Monday's. I take it seriously as part of my way of life, dedicating four hours to this, and it ensures a great week. After my house day, I complete and put away the laundry, which means my administrative work as household manager is complete for the week. I know some women do laundry all week with a constant pile of clothes on the table or couch where family time should be taking place. The invention of the washing machine allows laundry to be a side project, which is convenient, but it also allows you to put laundry in, then leave the house and forget about it.

What do I do with those thirty hours? I spend my thirty hours productively. I wash and gas my car once a week whether it needs it or not to ensure I don't ever run late if I'm low on gas. When I arrive at the car wash at 7:30 a.m., it only takes twenty minutes to get a car gassed and washed. If I go later in the day or on a weekend, it can take up to an hour. When I'm intentional with scheduling I feel I gain time. If you did the math, you know that doesn't add up to thirty hours. In fact, it's not even half of my weekly free time. In less than fifteen hours a week, I can have a clear head, a clean house, a workout, a shower, and dinner prepped every night. I still have fifteen hours a week to do whatever I want. Fridays are reserved for friendship day. I don't make any appointments or have any expectations, and I hang out with someone to do something fun. I look forward to laughing and carry the message not the mess.

They say to keep your spiritual fitness, you have to give it away. You've got to pass the torch. I can see how the preparation, visualization, time, team, and commitment prepared me for life after sports. Now is the time to share these values with my daughter. Softball brought me so much joy, even though it brought me pain as well.

There's a saying: Take what you need and leave the rest. I will pass on the joy of sports to my daughter and any others whom may cross my path, and I will leave the rest.

> "TAKE WHAT YOU NEED AND LEAVE THE REST."

Find something bigger than yourself and be a part of it. What can you visualize yourself doing to share your experience, strength, and hope? Do service work by sharing your talent with the youth or others. You only have to be one step ahead of someone to teach them. I believe you need a mentor—someone who has walked your path—and a mentee, someone you are guiding to stay tethered in the Holy Spirit.

CHAPTER 11
QUIT THE CHAOS

THE PEACEFUL WARRIOR

We will suddenly realize that God is doing for
us what we could not do for ourselves.

—*The Big Book*

A client approached me after she'd had her four kids. Now that her youngest was in kindergarten, she was ready to become her best self. She was interested in losing weight, learning healthy cooking habits, and raising an active family. She was middle-aged with wonderful kids and a husband who was successful. She was a kind and gentle spirit. Her husband's business was blooming, and because it was very public, she wanted to be her best self and not be held back by any insecurities in her appearance. I worked with her three days a week for two years. When she quickly got to her ideal body weight, she felt great. She learned the little tricks of the trade when it comes to making food choices. For example, have a green tea instead of a latte, eat well all week and enjoy a dinner out, and be conscious of drinking calories. Watching her come into herself was like watching a butterfly emerge from its cocoon. I am in awe of how she goes through life and keeps her sanity amidst all the moving parts of her family and business. She celebrates every milestone with her family. She puts her selfcare first, which makes her the best mother and wife. She retrained her brain to see the success in her days instead of the failures. She is winning every day, not only in the areas of food and fitness, but in her unwavering faith.

While coaching my daughter's recreational ten and under team or the junior high school team, whether we win or lose, standing on that field is a victory for me. I remember the selfish, unhappy, isolated, insecure, overweight person I used to be. Now, I share in the incremental victories with the girls and teach them character, healthy living, spiritual fitness, and hard work. I believe God put me on that field to show me He could put me anywhere. I knew I couldn't have gotten there without Him.

I track our wins not by the score book, but by how many girls return to the field year after year. I love it when a parent calls to let me know their daughter is making better food choices or understands that rest and recovery are just as important as training. My reward is when a client wants me to work with her daughter after she has been with me for many years. My favorite is when a mother brings her daughter who is getting ready for her bat mitzvah, quinceañera, or other rite of passage celebration. I get the chance to fill her up with positivity and help build her self-worth and self-image.

It's through the hardship of your journey that you accept that you were made to have a great life with spiritual connection. There are no mistakes, only lessons. To those of us who are moving in the self-awakening circles and consciousness movements, there is no shadow of a doubt that your fem is on the rise. According to Kingsbury, the Divine Feminine is the aspect of the self-associated with creation, intuition, community, sensuality (felt sense rather than thinking sense), and collaboration. No longer am I split in two by pain. I feel whole, and I embody spiritual fitness. I am love, and I am loved. I will be okay, no matter what. God is my source and my supply, not any person, place, or thing. The burden of expectations (of both myself and others) has been lifted. I can sift through the shit and say—*NO!* I have a voice. I am not searching to find myself. I am me, and I am love. I am a child of God, and I am imperfect just the way I am.

I am enough—We all face this self-limiting belief: I am not enough. No one is immune to the thought. It is what you do with it when it enters your head and your ability to overcome it with conviction that counts. You are enough just the way you are. You have been made with perfection by the Holy creator. You are exactly where you are supposed to be. Do the next right thing, and you will see the joy in life. What is your next best step?

I have enough—You will grow where you are planted. Having enough is a perspective. When you plant yourself in the Holy Spirit, you'll find He has given you everything you need to prosper. Don't wait for a new job, a new house, or a new spouse to be the best you can today. Just do the next best thing. When you feel a yearning to do something greater, the Holy Spirit is calling. Listen to the voice in your heart that is calling you for greatness. Don't delay—work with what you have.

WHERE THERE IS A WILL, THERE'S A WAY

I love my husband, my daughter, my family, and my friends in the best ways I know how, and I have also learned to love myself. It has taken a life time to believe that I deserve love and to remove the barriers of I am not enough, I don't have enough, I am not deserving, if only I was thinner, if only I was not afflicted—and all the other negative messages that played in my head. I can enjoy my everyday activities and see God working in the little things. I hope you can join me on the journey of self-reflection and spiritual enlightenment and be able to be kind to yourself and others. You experience the first creation once an idea pops in your mind. The second creation is manifesting the idea. Do not turn down the volume of your thoughts. When you have a thought, listen to your inner voice. When you have a will, the way will follow. As an athlete, I pictured myself in the batter's box hitting a home run. When game time arrived, I already hit the homerun twenty-five times over in my head. You must first picture the life you want and then follow up by taking action.

"Legacy is organizing the way you live your life so that you will be a blessing to people for generations to come. It is no more than taking the responsibility to ensure that your relationships and resources will outlive and outlast your time here on earth." Phil Munsey, *Legacy Now*.

Our lives can change in an instant. I am fortunate to be alive, and I want to live life to the fullest without regret and without hurting myself or others. Our calendars, and bodies don't lie, and neither will our obituaries. How we spend our precious time matters, so don't be prisoner to the jail cell between your ears. Master your mind and become a peaceful warrior. *Quitting to Win* is about making good decisions and making changes without fear. Leave a positive, uplifting, and peaceful legacy. Join the movement—*Quitting to Win!*

BIBLIOGRAPHY

Alcoholics Anonymous: The Story of How Many Thousands of Men and Women Have Recovered from Alcoholism. Alcoholics Anonymous World Services, 2001.

Burroughs, Stanley. *The Master Cleanser: with Special Needs and Problems.* Reno, NV: Burroughs Books, 2004.

Carney, Amy. *Parent on Purpose: A Courageous Approach to Raising Children in a Complicated World.* Niche Pressworks, 2019.

Chapman, Gary D. *The 5 Love Languages.* Northfield Pub., 2015.

Hepola, Sarah. *Blackout: Remembering the Things I Drank to Forget.* Two Roads, an Imprint of John Murray Press, 2016.

Kiyosaki, Robert T. *The Rich Dads Guide to Investing: What the Rich Invest in That the Poor Don't!* Scottsdale, AZ, 2012.

Leto, Kim Dolan. *F. I. T.: Faith, Inspired, Transformation.* Austin, TX: Fedd Books, 2014.

Mandarich, Tony, and Sharon Shaw. Elrod. *My Dirty Little Secrets-- Steroids, Alcohol & God: the Tony Mandarich Story.* Modern History Press, 2009.

Melton, Glennon Doyle. *Love Warrior.* MacMillan USA, 2017.

Munsey, Phil. *Legacy Now.* Lake Mary, FL: Charisma House, 2008.

Oberbrunner, Kary. *Your Secret Name: An Uncommon Quest to Stop Pretending, Shed the Labels, and Discover Your True Identity.* Author Academy Elite, 2018.

Websites

Alcoholics Anonymous. "Many Paths to Spirituality." www.aa.org/assets/en_US/p-84_manypathstospirituality.pdf

Bustillos, Esteban. "The Lifelong Impact of Sports on Girls and Women." www.wbgh.com. (accessed December 9, 2019).

"Common Suicide Warning Signs." https://www.doctoroz.com/article/common-suicide-warning-signs (accessed March 4, 2020).

Dictionary.com https://www.dictionary.com (accessed March 4, 2020).

Harvard Health Publishing. "Suicide survivors face grief, questions, challenges." Https://www.health.harvard.edu/blog/suicide-survivors-face-grief-questions-challenges-201408127342 (accessed August 12, 2014).

Kingsbury, Suzanne. "The Divine Feminine founder of Gateless Writing."

National Institute of Arthritis and Musculoskeletal and Skin Diseases. "What People Recovering From Alcoholism Need To Know About Osteoporosis." https://www.bones.nih.gov/health-info/bone/osteoporosis/conditions-behaviors/alcoholism (accessed March 4, 2020).

Acronyms

LOVE:
Let
Others
Voluntarily
Evolve

EGO:
Edging
God
Out.

HALT:
Don't get too:
Hungry
Angry
Lonely
Tired

QTIP:
Quit
Taking
It
Personally

APPENDIX I

SUICIDE RESOURCES

Signs of Suicide

- Sadness

- Depression

- Low self-worth

- Feeling hopeless or trapped

- Decreased or increased appetite

- Sleeping too much or too little

- Pulling away from family and friends; isolating oneself

- Lack of interest in things that once were enjoyable

- Increased drug and alcohol use

- Mood swings

- Focusing on death – talking, reading or writing about it

Suicide Grief

Did you know? The grief process is always difficult. But a loss through suicide is like no other, and grieving can be especially complex and traumatic. People coping with this kind of loss often need more support than others but may get less. (https://www.health.harvard.edu/blog/ suicide-survivors-face-grief-questions-challenges-201408127342)

Suicide Resources

If you or a loved one is exhibiting any of these warning signs, there are resources that can help:

- National Suicide Prevention Lifeline: 800-273-8255
- American Foundation for Suicide Prevention
- Crisis Text Line: Text HOME to 741-741
- Veterans Crisis Line
- American Psychiatric Association

APPENDIX II

MORE IN-DEPTH QUESTIONS AND ANSWERS TO THE TWELVE QUESTIONS.

Answer YES or NO to the following twelve questions.

1. Have you ever decided to stop drinking for a week or so, but only lasted for a couple of days?

Most of us in A.A. made all kinds of promises to ourselves and to our families. We could not keep them. Then we came to A.A. A.A. said: "Just try not to drink today." (If you do not drink today, you cannot get drunk today.)

Yes No

2. Do you wish people would mind their own business about your drinking-- stop telling you what to do?

In A.A. we do not tell anyone to do anything. We just talk about our own drinking, the trouble we got into, and how we stopped. We will be glad to help you, if you want us to.

Yes No

3. Have you ever switched from one kind of drink to another in the hope that this would keep you from getting drunk?

We tried all kinds of ways. We made our drinks weak. Or just drank beer. Or we did not drink cocktails. Or only drank on weekends. You name it; we tried it. But if we drank anything with alcohol in it, we usually got drunk eventually.

Yes No

4. Have you had to have an eye-opener upon awakening during the past year?

Do you need a drink to get started or to stop shaking? This is a pretty sure sign that you are not drinking *socially*.

Yes No

5. Do you envy people who can drink without getting into trouble?

At one time or another, most of us have wondered why we were not like most people, who really can take it or leave it.

Yes No

6. Have you had problems connected with drinking during the past year?

Be honest! Doctors say that if you have a problem with alcohol and keep on drinking, it will get worse, never better. Eventually, you will die or end up in an institution for the rest of your life. The only hope is to stop drinking.

Yes No

7. Has your drinking caused trouble at home?

Before we came into A.A., most of us said that it was the people or problems at home that made us drink. We could not see that our drinking just made everything worse. It never solved problems anywhere or anytime.

Yes No

8. Do you ever try to get "extra" drinks at a party because you do not get enough?

Most of us used to have a *few* before we started out if we thought it was going to be that kind of party. And if drinks were not served fast enough, we would go someplace else to get more.

Yes No

9. Do you tell yourself you can stop drinking any time you want to, even though you keep getting drunk when you don't mean to?

Many of us kidded ourselves into thinking that we drank because we wanted to. After we came into A.A., we found out once we started to drink, we couldn't stop.

Yes No

10. Have you missed days of work or school because of drinking?

Many of us admit now that we called in sick lots of times when the truth was that we were hung-over or drunk.

Yes No

11. Do you have "blackouts"?

A blackout is when we have been drinking hours or days and cannot remember. When we came to A.A., we found out that this is a pretty sure sign of alcoholic drinking.

Yes No

12. Have you ever felt that your life would be better if you did not drink?

Many of us started to drink because drinking made life seem better, at least for a while. By the time we got into A.A., we felt trapped. We were drinking to live and living to drink. We were sick and tired of being sick and tired.

Yes No

RESULTS

Did you answer **YES** four or more times? If so, you are probably
in trouble with alcohol. Why do we say this? Because thousands
of people in A.A. have said so for many years. They found out
the truth about themselves—the hard way. But again, only *you*
can decide whether you think A.A. is for you. Try to keep an
open mind on the subject. If the answer is **YES,** we will be glad
to show you how we stopped drinking ourselves. Just call. A.A.
does not promise to solve your life›s problems. But we can show
you how we are learning to live without drinking «one day at a
time.» We stay away from that first drink. If there is no first one,
there cannot be a tenth one. And when we got rid of alcohol, we
found that life became much more manageable.

ALCOHOLICS ANONYMOUS© is a fellowship of men and
women who share their experience, strength and hope with each
other that they may solve their common problem and help others
to recover from alcoholism.

- The only requirement for membership is a desire
  to stop drinking. There are no dues or fees for A.A.
  membership; we are self-supporting through our own
  contributions.

- A.A. is not allied with any sect, denomination, politics,
  organization or institution; does not wish to engage
  in any controversy; neither endorses nor opposes any
  causes.

- Our primary purpose is to stay sober and help other
  alcoholics to achieve sobriety.

Copyright © by The A.A. Grapevine, Inc.;
reprinted with permission

If you need help: http://www.aa.org/
SAMHSA- Substance Abuse and Mental Service Administration
-Health Hotline 1-800-662-HELP (4257)

APPENDIX II

Common Big Book Slogans

- Easy does it.
- First things first.
- Live and let live.
- But for the grace of God.
- Let go and let God.
- This too shall pass.
- Keep coming back ... it works if you work it.
- Stick with the winners.
- Sobriety is a journey ... not a destination.
- Faith without works is dead.
- If God seems far away, who moved?
- Turn it over.
- We are only as sick as our secrets.
- There are no coincidences in AA.
- Be part of the solution, not the problem.
- I can't handle it, God, you take over.
- One hour at a time.
  One day at a time.
  One step at a time
- Wonderful things happen.
  One Day At A Time
- Keep an open mind.
- Willingness is the key.
- More will be revealed.

- You will intuitively know.

- Don't quit 5 minutes before the miracle happens.

- Some of us are sicker than others.

- Alcoholism is an equal opportunity destroyer.

- Practice an attitude of gratitude.

- The road to sobriety is a simple journey for confused people with a complicated disease.

- God is never late.

- Have a good day unless, of course. you have made other plans.

- 90 meetings in 90 days ... 90/90.

- I can have complete serenity at this very moment ... if I live in denial.

- We came to AA to save our ass and found out our soul was attached.

- It's alcohol-ISM, not alcohol-WASM!

- I can only carry the message; I can't carry the drunk!

- Seven missed meetings makes one weak.

- Don't take everything personally.

APPENDIX III
DISCUSSION QUESTIONS

Chapter 1 Quit Wishing It Was You and Not Them
Do you or a loved one need to deal with a mental illness?

Chapter 2 Quit Wishing You Had Someone Else's Life
What story will you share with a confidant to release the shame and guilt? Can you accept your past and heal yourself?

Chapter 3 Quit Taking the Edge Off
Are there people in your life that are toxic?
Do you feel filled up or drained when you leave a friend?
Are you hanging out with the chickens, or soaring with the eagles?

Chapter 4 Quit the Insanity
Surrender: What are you doing that is holding you back from being your best self? Should you consider stopping the drink, or other bad habits?
I will stop … fill in the blank.
Do I need a support group or coach to show me how to change everything?

Chapter 5 Quit Sitting on the Pedestal
Have you gotten away from what healed you?
What do you need to do to avoid a bad habit relapse?

Chapter 6 Quit Using Other People's Versions of God
What prayer will you add to your day?
Write it here.

Chapter 7 Quit Depending on Others for Your Joy
Do you believe happiness is a choice?
When was the last time you thought of yourself as a victim?
Now take a step back and ask yourself what was God doing for you that you could not do for yourself?

Chapter 8 Quit Eating Empty Calories
What can you quit immediately that will reduce inflammation?
Which one of my favorite plant-based recipes will you try this week? What days will you go meat free?
What day will you do food prep for the week?

Chapter 9 Quit Running Someone Else's Race
Are you in physical pain?
Does it affect your daily living?
Start a journal to document how and when discomfort arrives.
What morning stretch will you add first thing in the morning?
Do you want to start the discovery process with an expert to see what is happening?
Who will you schedule an appointment with?

Chapter 10 Quit Turning off Your Inner Voice
What lesson in life did you learn early on that you are good at?

Chapter 11 Quit the Chaos
Are you at peace with yourself?
Do you show up on time and prepared?

Join the Movement

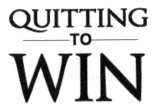

Your Next Steps start with
Quitting to Win Courses

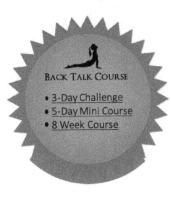

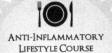

BACK TALK COURSE

- 3-Day Challenge
- 5-Day Mini Course
- 8 Week Course

ANTI-INFLAMMATORY
LIFESTYLE COURSE

- 3-Day Challenge
- 5-Day Mini Course
- 8 Week Course

CrystalWaltman.com

QUITTING
—TO—
WIN

Bring Crystal into your Organization

Are you looking for a dynamic speaker? Do you want a presentation for your groups need?

Crystal knows the importance of selecting the best speaker for your setting.

She speaks to organizations, companies, and women's groups about personal growth, communication, leadership, and becoming the people they were designed to be. From classrooms and boardrooms, to ballrooms and camp settings. She can lead workshops, for churches or corporate events.

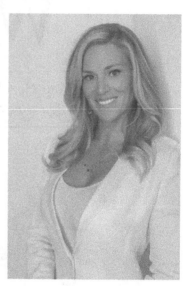

CrystalWaltman.com

Her engagements are centered on helping women take off their masks, live untamed and spiritually fit. Her message will connect with every individual in the room.

Crystal customizes her signature message to exceed each client's objectives.

Author—Speaker—Coach

ABOUT THE PUBLISHER

Do you dream of becoming an author? Want to share your message with the world? Publishing a book the right way can bring you more freedom, finances, and fulfillment. Meet my publisher.

This has truly been a great experience for me every step of the way.

Kary Oberbrunner with Author Academy shows you insider tips and tools on how to write, publish, and market your book successfully. Receive a FREE Author Guidebook when you register below.

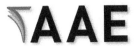

HTTPS://TINYURL.COM/CRYSTALWALTMAN

CPSIA information can be obtained
at www.ICGtesting.com
Printed in the USA
FSHW012234070720